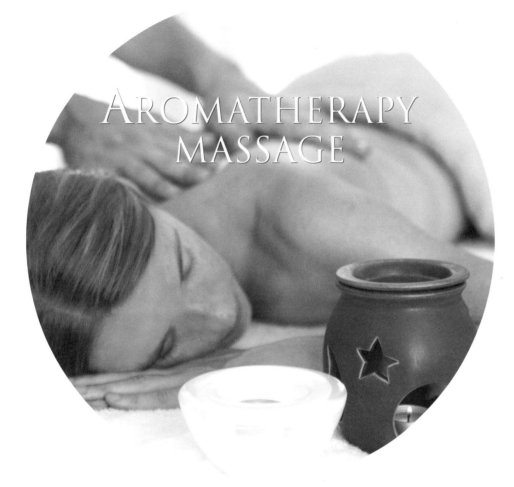

AROMATHERAPY MASSAGE

AROMATHERAPY MASSAGE

Essential oils explained for health and pleasure

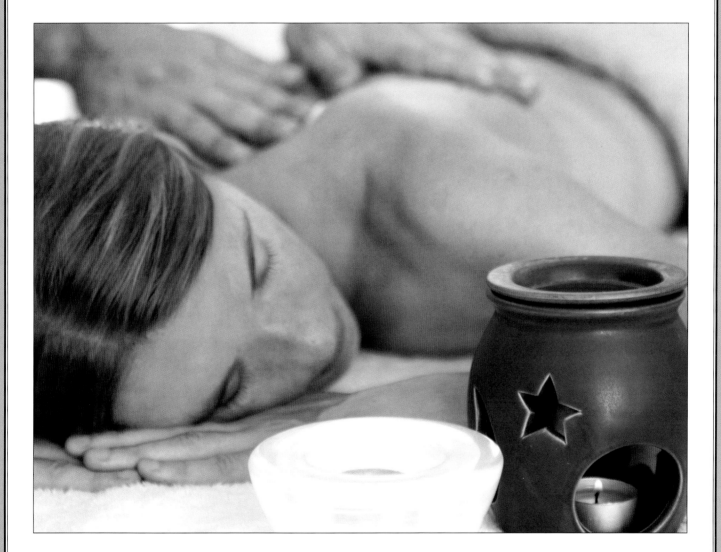

HINKLER BOOKS

MARGIE HARE

Art Director: Karen Moores
Editor: Margaret Barca
Design: Susie Allen
Photographer: Glenn Weiss
Special thanks to Mud Brick Herb Cottage
and also to Lee-Ann Dixon and Rock O'Keefe

First published in 2004
by Hinkler Books Pty Ltd
17-23 Redwood Drive
Dingley Victoria 3172 Australia
www.hinklerbooks.com

© Hinkler Books Pty Ltd 2004

All rights reserved.
No part of this publication may be reproduced or utilised in any form
or by any means electronic or mechanical, including photocopying,
recording or by any information storage or retrieval system now
known or hereafter invented, without the prior written permission of
Hinkler Books Pty Ltd.

Printed and bound in China

ISBN 1 7412 1635 4

The Publishers and their respective employees or agents, will not accept
responsibility for injury or damage occasioned to any person as a result of
participation in the activities described in this book.

CONTENTS

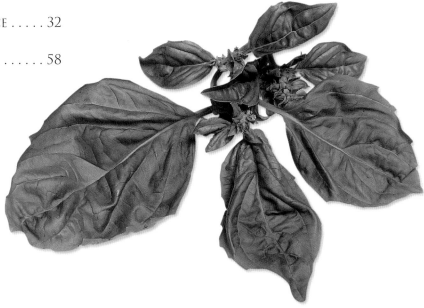

WHAT IS AROMATHERAPY?

Aromatherapy is a healing therapy that utilises the properties and aromas of essential plant oils. When we 'take time to smell the roses', there may be more to it than we think. Rose essential oil has many properties – it is an antidepressant, antiseptic, anti-spasmodic, antiviral, aphrodisiac, astringent, bactericide, laxative, sedative and heart tonic, to mention a few.

Aromatherapy uses pure essential oils skilfully and in a controlled manner to influence mind, body and soul for physical and emotional health and wellbeing. The modern usage of the word 'aromatherapie' originated with the French chemist René Maurice Gattefosse. In the 1920s he suffered burns to his arm and hand in a laboratory accident. He plunged his arm into a container of pure lavender essential oil, mistaking it for water. Despite third degree burns he made a speedy recovery with no scarring. He subsequently researched the properties of lavender that caused this recovery and passed his findings on to the medical profession. During World War II, lavender oil was used to help save soldiers' limbs that were being lost to gangrene.

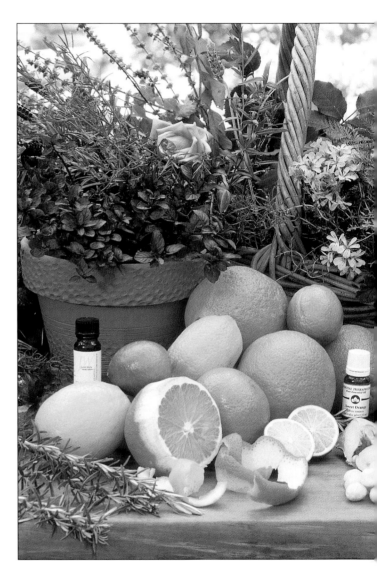

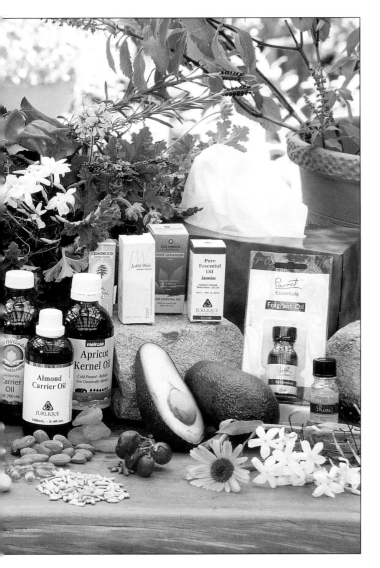

THE HISTORY OF AROMATHERAPY

The use of plants, aromas and natural ingredients for healing and improving health dates back thousands of years. Essential oils were used by the ancient civilisations of Egypt, China, the Middle East, India and Greece.

In Egypt, exotic perfumes were used in abundance by the Pharaohs and their families.

Oils were used in embalming and in the temples they were used as offerings to the gods. The Greeks and the Romans were famous for the use of aromatic oils and massage in their bath houses. In the Middle East plants were used widely for their medicinal and therapeutic properties. Oils and aromatic medicines were brought to Europe from the Middle East by the crusaders. Aromatherapy developed during the Middle Ages in Europe into one of the most sought after forms of natural healing. In Asia the oldest form of Indian medicine is known as Ayurvedic, and an important aspect of this principle is massage with essential oils.

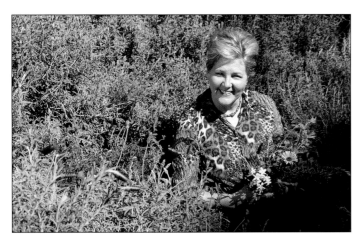

The author, Margie Hare

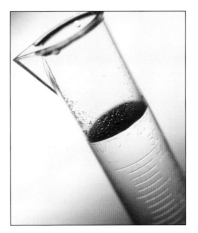

WHAT IS AROMATHERAPY?

(continued)

WHAT ARE ESSENTIAL OILS?

Essential oils occur widely in the plant kingdom and are sometimes referred to as the plants' 'life force'. They are minute drops of liquid occurring in glands, hairs or veins of flowers, leaves, seeds, bark and wood, resin, roots or fruit peel of the plant. They give the plant its very specific scent. These droplets are a mixture of complex, organic compounds. When extracted they are highly concentrated and volatile (which means that they turn quickly from a liquid into a gas at room temperature and higher). In lavender they occur in the flowering tops of lavender, in oranges in the peel and in rosemary in the leaves. The most common form of extraction is by steam distillation.

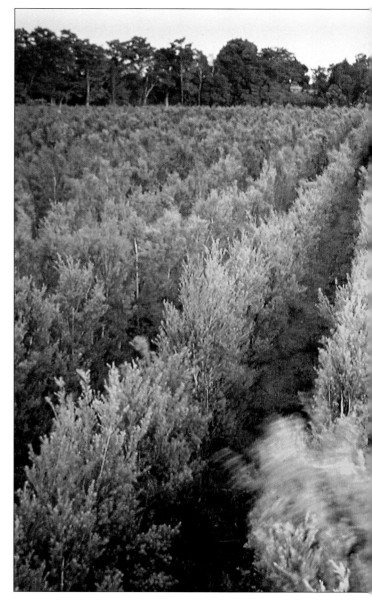

Main Camp Tea Tree Oil Distillation Plant, Northern NSW
Photo courtesy of TP Health Ltd, Ballina NSW

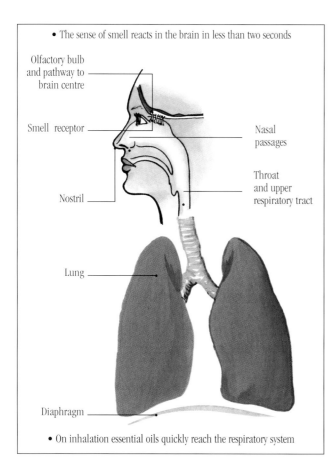

• The sense of smell reacts in the brain in less than two seconds

Olfactory bulb and pathway to brain centre

Smell receptor

Nasal passages

Throat and upper respiratory tract

Nostril

Lung

Diaphragm

• On inhalation essential oils quickly reach the respiratory system

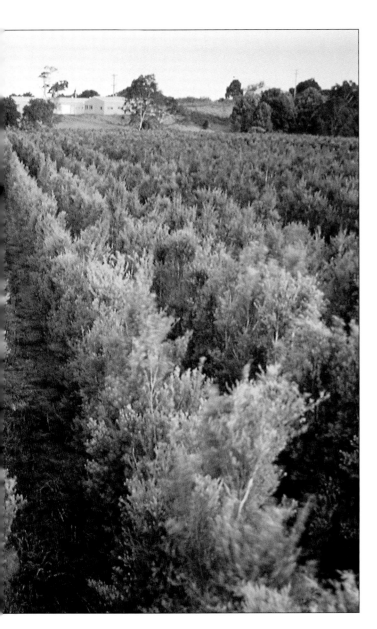

HOW ESSENTIAL OILS WORK

Essential oils enter the body by two main routes – the skin and the nose. They enter and leave the body efficiently, leaving no toxins behind. When inhaled, essential oils come into contact with the olfactory system located in the nose and behind the eyes. These oils are also absorbed easily through the pores and hair follicles in the skin. Essential oils are taken directly into the blood stream; they have a positive effect on blood circulation, helping to bring oxygen and nutrients to the tissues whilst assisting in the disposal of carbon dioxide and other waste materials.

I believe aromatherapy works in a holistic way addressing the mind, body and soul. The main benefits come from the pleasant fragrances, which have a positive psychological effect.

There are so many pure essential oils to choose from. Here is just a selection.

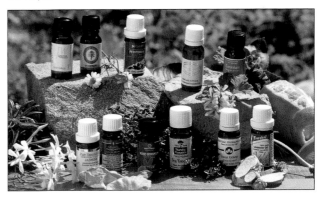

GUIDELINES WHEN USING ESSENTIAL OILS

Essential oils are highly concentrated. It is important to follow the dosages recommended. More is not better. On the contrary, it can have an adverse effect. The difference in the effect between one drop and two drops can be substantial.

GENERAL CAUTIONS

- Do not take internally
- Keep out of reach of children
- Avoid using essential oils near eyes and other sensitive areas
- Always read the precautions on the bottle before using
- Use only 100% pure essential oils
- Keep oils away from any naked flame
- Store oils well sealed in a cool, dark place
- Never use neat (except where indicated, see page 68).

Some oils can increase the risk of sunburn

SPECIAL CAUTIONS

- Avoid the following essential oils during pregnancy: basil, cedar aurantiumwood, clary sage, clove bud, cypress, fennel, jasmine, juniper, lemongrass, marjoram, peppermint, rosemary, thyme.
- Do not use essential oils on newborn babies.
- Some oils can cause photo-sensitisation of the skin, increasing the risk of sunburn. These include bergamot, ginger, lemon, lemon verbena, lime, mandarin and orange.
- The following oils should not be used on sensitive skins: basil, fennel, lemongrass, lemon, lemon verbena, melissa, orange, peppermint, thyme.
- Avoid sage, thyme, cypress and rosemary oil if there is any possibility of high blood pressure, epilepsy or kidney disease.
- If having to drive a long distance after a massage, do not use clary sage, marjoram or ylang ylang – they can cause drowsiness.
- If prone to epilepsy do not use fennel, rosemary or sage.

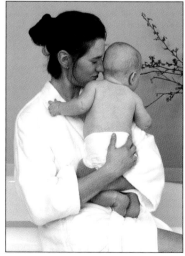

Essential oils can be used safely on babies. See page 75.

BENEFITS OF AROMATHERAPY MASSAGE

The purpose of aromatherapy massage is to aid the penetration of essential oils into the body and to treat problem areas. Massage can be stimulating or relaxing depending on the oils used and the technique applied. It is an effective way to relieve stress, anxiety and tension. Aromatherapy massage combines the balancing properties of the essential oils with the relaxing benefits of touch. As the oils are absorbed into the skin and the muscles relax, the therapeutic benefits manifest. Psychologically, massage promotes a wonderful feeling of lightness and wellbeing. Massage is a valuable gift to give a friend – it not only soothes the mind and body but it has numerous other benefits. A good aromatherapy massage will:

- increase metabolism
- speed up the healing process
- enhance the removal of toxins
- increase muscle and joint mobility
- improve skin tone
- aid relaxation by calming the nervous system
- improve circulation of blood and lymph
- relieve mental and physical tiredness
- reduce aches, pains, spasms and stiffness
- improve digestion.

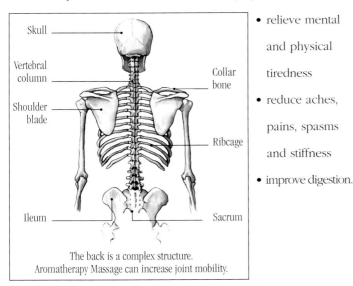

The back is a complex structure.
Aromatherapy Massage can increase joint mobility.

Skull

Vertebral column

Shoulder blade

Collar bone

Ribcage

Ileum

Sacrum

Deltoid

Trapezius

Latissimus dorsi

Forearm extensors

Gluteus maximus

Hamstrings

Gastrocnemius

Achilles tendon

Orbicularis ori

Orbicularis

Platysma

Pectoralis major

Biceps brachii

Rectus abdominus

Quadriceps

Sartorus

Tibialis anterior

The muscle system: Be aware of the muscle structure as you massage. Muscles become more flexible and muscle tension and cramps are reduced during massage.

GETTING STARTED

This book is not intended to enable you to treat the public professionally or to replace your general practitioner. It is intended to give you the confidence to use essential oils safely, have fun, treat your friends and family and enjoy the wonderful benefits of aromatherapy in the home. Treat simple everyday ailments, but if they persist or become severe seek professional help.

MEASUREMENTS

Useful information when working with essential oils

- 20 drops = 1 ml essential oil
- 1 ml essential oil = 1 cc
- 10 ml bottle contains 200 drops
- 100 drops = 1 teaspoon = 5 cc

ESSENTIALS IN YOUR STARTER KIT

- stainless steel/enamel/china footbath
- 1 box Epsom/Dead Sea salts
- 1 bottle sweet almond carrier oil
- 9 essential oils: lavender, tea tree, peppermint, chamomile, eucalyptus, geranium, rosemary, lemon, orange
- 1 jar vegetable base cream
- glass measuring cylinder
- stainless steel stirrer
- selection of empty dark glass bottles and jars

Aromatherapy starter kits may be ordered at
www.divinearomatherapy.com.au

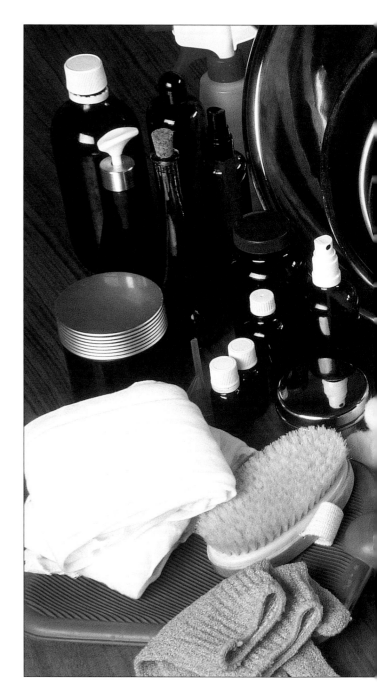

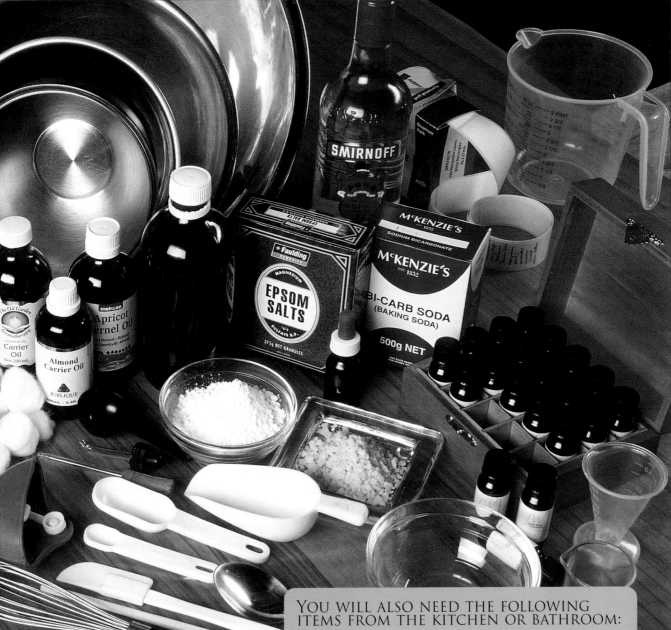

You will also need the following items from the kitchen or bathroom:

- stainless steel mixing bowls and whisk
- a teaspoon and a tablespoon measure
- tissues
- spatula
- 1 litre bottled spring/filtered water
- glycerin
- full cream milk/cream/powdered goats' milk
- hot water bottle
- towels
- paper towel
- cottonwool, cleansing pads and cottonbuds
- nip of vodka
- honey
- rice flour or cornflour
- blank labels

POPULAR AROMATHERAPY OILS

Essential oils are derived from leaves, flowers, roots, the peel of certain fruits and other parts of aromatic plants. Hundreds of plants have been used over the centuries for medicinal and therapeutic purposes and for general well-being. Modern aromatherapy uses a more limited selection, though their effects are wide-ranging.

This is not a complete reference for all essential oils, but is a selection of some of the most popular and safest oils for home use.

Study the guide and refer to it before using your essential oils.

In particular, be aware of any special cautions advised.

BASIL
THE APHRODISIAC OIL

Botanical name *Ocimum basilicum*

Plant part used Flowering sweet basil tops and leaves.

Main benefits Used for nervous insomnia, anxiety and tiredness. Helpful for insect bites, headaches, muscular aches and pains.

Blending suggestions Blends well with eucalyptus, frankincense, geranium, ginger, lavender, lemon, rosemary, peppermint, pine, thyme and tea tree.

My comment Use in hair conditioning treatment.

Cautions Avoid during pregnancy. Use with caution on sensitive skin as it can be an irritant.

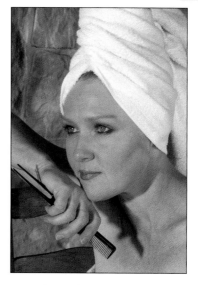

Use as a hair conditioning treatment

BERGAMOT
THE UPLIFTING OIL

Botanical name

Citrus aurantium

Plant part used

Peel of the bitter orange.

Main benefits Good for relaxing tight, aching muscles.

Blending suggestions For massage, bergamot is extremely versatile and can lift any blend. Try it with marjoram, jasmine and rose or sandalwood.

My comment Try bergamot neat on cold sores as well as in uplifting body freshening spray.

Cautions Do not use when going in the sun.

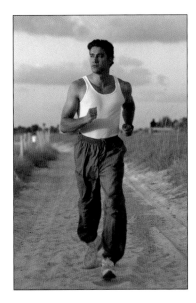

Use for athlete's foot

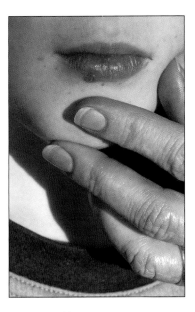

Use to treat cold sores

CEDARWOOD (ATLAS)
A REFRESHING OIL FOR MEN

Botanical name *Cedrus atlantica*

Main benefits This oil has a stimulating, refreshing and tonic effect on the body. It is good for dandruff, eczema, greasy skin and acne. It is an effective insect repellent.

Blending suggestions This oil blends well with bergamot, cypress, frankincense, juniper, lavender, rosemary and lemon.

My comment Use for athlete's foot.

Cautions Avoid during pregnancy. This oil should be avoided by breast-feeding mothers and by children.

POPULAR AROMATHERAPY OILS

(continued)

CHAMOMILE (ROMAN)
THE SOOTHING OIL

Botanical name

Chamaemelum nobile

Plant part used

Freshly dried flowers.

Main benefits This oil is a natural
anti-inflammatory with great healing properties as well as
relaxing sedative benefits.

Blending suggestions Chamomile is an expensive oil
and you can substitute some drops with lavender when
using to ease pain. Blends well with geranium, lavender,
patchouli and rose.

My comment Safe for use on babies, children and pets.

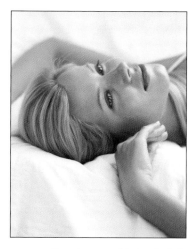

Promotes a peaceful state of mind

CLARY SAGE
THE ANTIDEPRESSANT OIL

Botanical name

Salvia sclarea

Plant part used

Leaves and flowers.

Main benefits

Calming, promotes a peaceful state of mind and restful
sleep, improves mental clarity and alertness, and reduces
stress and tension.

Blending suggestions Blends well with cedarwood,
geranium, juniper, lavender and sandalwood.

My comment Use in massage oil blend for varicose
veins.

Cautions This essential oil should not be used in large
doses, as it can be stupefying. Clary sage is well known
for its euphoric action. Not to be used during pregnancy.

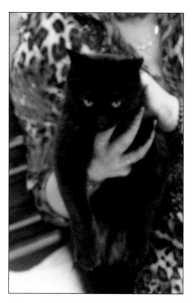

Safe to use on animals

EUCALYPTUS
THE PERFECT INSECT REPELLENT

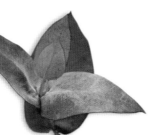

Botanical name

Eucalyptus globulus

Plant part used

Fresh leaves and twigs.

Main benefits Because eucalyptus oil prevents bacterial growth and inhibits the growth of viruses it is used to treat burns, blisters, cuts, herpes, wounds and sores. Has been used for centuries by Aboriginal communities for healing wounds. Added to massage oil, cream and baths it soothes the pain of sore muscles, arthritis and rheumatism.

Blending suggestions The clean camphor-like perfume of eucalyptus blends well with lavender, rosemary, tea tree and pine.

My comment Gargle and steam-inhalation for sore throats and persistent coughs.

Cautions Avoid using this oil if suffering from high blood pressure or epilepsy. Do not use this oil whilst on homoeopathic remedies – it could negate the healing effect. Do not take internally.

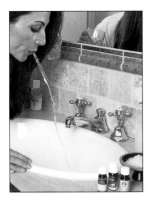

Use as a gargle for sore throat

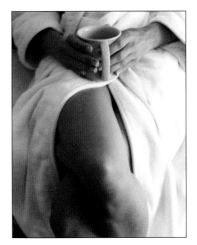

Helps reduce cellulite deposits

GERANIUM
THE WOMEN'S OIL

Botanical name

Pelargonium graveolens

Plant part used

Leaves and flowers.

Main benefits Geranium oil has a regulatory action on the hormones secreted by the adrenal cortex. Ideal for PMT and menopause. It reduces stress and tension, is calming and uplifting, speeds body healing, eases depression and is helpful in managing asthma. It also acts as a tonic and diuretic on the urinary system and the liver, which helps rid the body of toxins.

Blending suggestions Geranium's relaxing, rose-scented, heady aroma blends well and balances most other fragrances.

My comment Use in a massage blend to help reduce cellulite deposits.

Cautions Dilute further than standard dosage on sensitive skins as it may cause irritation. Avoid long-term use with history of oestrogen-dependant cancer.

POPULAR AROMATHERAPY OILS

(continued)

GINGER
THE WARMING OIL

Botanical name

Zingiber officinale

Plant part used Rhizome.

Main benefits A warming oil that relaxes tight muscles, relieves aches and pains, making it a natural choice to treat arthritis. Useful in the treatment of cold and coughs. Also improves digestion as it stimulates the gastric juices.

Blending suggestions The rich, spicy perfume of ginger blends well with lavender, lemon, grapefruit, orange and petitgrain.

My comment Try as a chest rub for the winter chills.

Cautions Do not use on open skin. May cause irritation. Do not use within 72 hours of going into the sun.

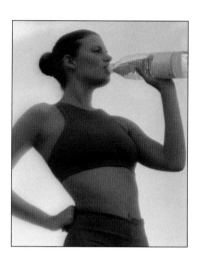

For an uplifting and reviving effect
— use in massage blend

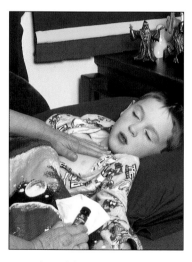

Try as chest rub for winter chills

GRAPEFRUIT
THE CELLULITE OIL

Botanical name

Citrus paradisi

Plant part used

Fruit rind.

Main benefits This oil has an uplifting and reviving effect, making it useful in treating stress, depression and nervous exhaustion. Grapefruit is a lymphatic stimulant, so it is helpful in the treatment of water retention as well as having fat-dissolving properties.

Blending suggestions This fresh, sweet citrus aroma blends well with basil, bergamot, cedarwood, ginger, lime, lavender, rosemary and ylang ylang.

Cautions A very safe oil to use. It is non-toxic, non-irritant and will not make the skin sensitive to the sun.

JASMINE
THE ROMANTIC OIL

Botanical name

Jasminum grandiflorum

Plant part used

Fresh flowers.

Main benefits

Uplifting, relaxing and an excellent brain stimulant. It is good for dry sensitive skins and to treat muscular aches and menstrual cramps.

Blending suggestions This exotic, rich aroma blends well with lavender, orange, mandarin, neroli, rose, rosewood and sandalwood.

My comment Always use this oil to lighten the emotional load.

Cautions Non-toxic, non-irritant. Not to be used during pregnancy.

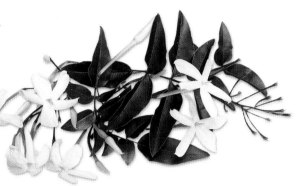

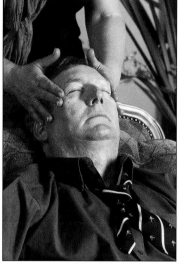

Great for treating migraines

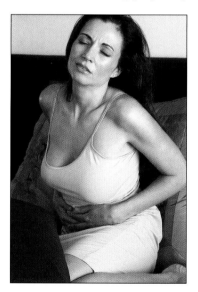

For relief of menstrual cramps

LAVENDER
ESSENTIAL OIL FOR THE FIRST AID KIT

Botanical name

Lavandula angustifolia

Plant part used

Fresh flowers.

Main benefits Lavender is well known for its sedative properties and is useful in treating depression, migraine, insomnia and nervous tension as well as dealing with stress.

Blending suggestions The floral, sweet scent of lavender blends well with bergamot, clary sage, lemon, mandarin, orange, pine, rosemary and ylang ylang.

My comment Use neat on burns and even sunburn.

Cautions Non-toxic, non-irritant. Not suitable for very young children

POPULAR AROMATHERAPY OILS

(continued)

LEMON
THE CLEANSING OIL

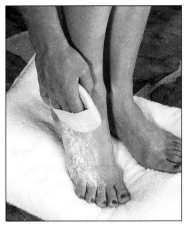

Use as an anti-fungal foot powder

Botanical name *Citrus limon*

Plant part used Rind of fruit.

Main benefits Lemon is stimulating, invigorating, astringent, deodorising and antiseptic. Very helpful in treating mental exhaustion. Also for energising an aching body. Used in the treatment of cellulite.

Blending suggestions The tangy, fresh citrus aroma blends with bergamot, eucalyptus, frankincense, ginger, juniper, lavender, rose and rosemary.

My comment Use in facial steam for normal skin.

Cautions Do not use this oil within 72 hours of going into the sun.

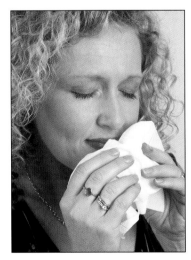

Use in tissue inhalation to
stimulate and invigorate

LEMONGRASS
THE REGENERATIVE OIL

Botanical name

Cymbopogon flexuosus

Plant part used Fresh and partially dried fronds.

Main benefits A good tonic for the skin, especially useful for athlete's foot. Lemongrass kills bacteria and fungal infections. It cools and reduces fever in the body and helps ease aching muscles. Lemongrass calms the nervous system relieving depression, stress and nervous exhaustion.

Blending suggestions The warm, lemon, grassy aroma blends well with cedarwood, geranium, jasmine, lavender, neroli, rosemary and tea tree.

My comment Good oil for fungal infections.

Cautions Use with care on sensitive skins – it can cause irritation due to high citrus content. Not suitable for toddlers. Halve the adult dilution as recommended for all topical applications. Use only 3 drops in the bath. Not to be used during pregnancy.

LIME
THE UPLIFTING OIL

Botanical name

Citrus aurantifolia

Plant part used

Fruit peel.

Main benefits This oil is antibacterial, antifungal and antiseptic. A great stimulant and tonic. Very useful for treating colds and flu, cellulite, poor circulation, greasy skin, arthritis and varicose veins.

Blending suggestions The sweet, fresh fragrance of the lime blends well with bergamot, cedarwood, geranium, grapefruit, lavender, lemon, mandarin, neroli, orange, rosemary, vetiver and ylang ylang.

My comment Uplifting oil for bath and massage when feeling tired.

Cautions Can cause sensitivity. This oil is photo-sensitive. Do not use within 72 hours of going into the sun.

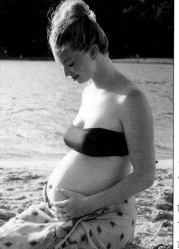

Use in massage blend to reduce stretch marks during pregnancy

Photo by Theresa Jamieson

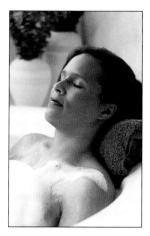

Use in a bath when feeling tired

MANDARIN
THE CHILDREN'S OIL

Botanical name

Citrus reticulata

Plant part used

Fruit peel.

Main benefits

Having great digestive properties, it relieves cramps, spasms and stimulates bile production. It also aids digestion, constipation and hiccoughs. A great oil to use for stretch marks, scars and aging skin.

Blending suggestions The citrus, sweet floral perfume of lime blends well with basil, bergamot, chamomile, grapefruit, lavender, lemon, neroli, orange, petitgrain and rose.

My comment Use this oil during pregnancy to help reduce stretch marks.

Cautions Non-toxic and non-irritant. This oil can be photo-sensitive. Do not use within 72 hours of going in the sun.

POPULAR AROMATHERAPY OILS

(continued)

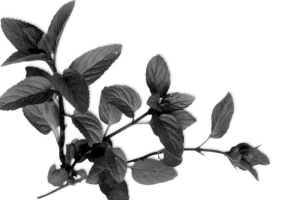

MARJORAM
THE CALMING OIL

Botanical name

Origanum majorana

Plant part used Flowering tops and leaves.

Main benefits Marjoram relieves tight muscles, aches and pains, reduces inflammation, improves digestion and helps relieve congestion.

Blending suggestions The woody, spicy and camphor-like aroma blends well with bergamot, cedarwood, chamomile, clary sage, cypress, eucalyptus, juniper, lavender, mandarin, patchouli, rosemary and tea tree.

My comment Use in bath and massage oil to calm and sedate.

Cautions Avoid during pregnancy. Avoid if you suffer from low blood pressure.

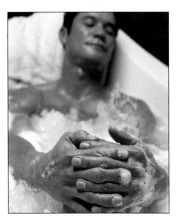

Use in a bath to calm and sedate

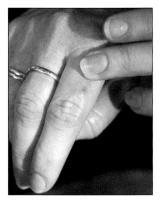

Soothes and relieves insect stings

MELISSA
THE HEART OIL

Botanical name

Melissa officinalis

Plant part used Flowering tops and leaves.

Main benefits Melissa calms and soothes the skin (eczema, acne and insect stings) as well as soothing the mind by calming the nervous system (grief, depression, sadness and stress). Respiratory-related allergies (hayfever, asthma and skin reactions) respond well to melissa. Melissa offers relief for problems of the digestive or circulatory system (slows heart palpitations, lowers blood pressure, eases headaches and migraine, calms a persistent cough).

Blending suggestions Its sweet, gentle, lemon aroma blends well with basil, bergamot, chamomile, frankincense, geranium, ginger, lavender, neroli, rosemary and ylang ylang.

My comment Relax in the bath with 6–8 drops of this calming oil.

Cautions Avoid during pregnancy. There is a risk of allergic reaction due to the high aldehyde content. Use in weaker dilution.

NEROLI

THE MIND, BODY AND SOUL OIL

Botanical name *Citrus aurantium*

Plant part used Fresh flowers.

Main benefits It helps prevent wrinkles, stretch marks and thread veins. It has a deep tranquillising effect and is used for treating anxiety, depression, palpitations and nervous disorders. The digestive properties of neroli relieve diarrhoea, indigestion, cramps and spasms and help expel gas from the intestines.

Blending suggestions The exquisite sweet perfume of this oil blends well with most other oils.

My comment Inhale on a tissue or add two drops to your pillow to relieve insomnia.

Cautions Safe and ideal to use during pregnancy.

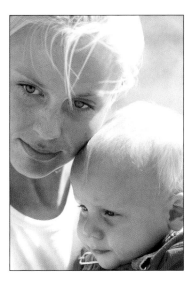

Excellent oil for calming children

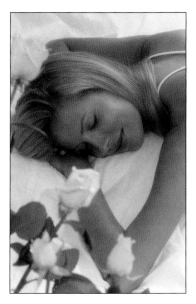

Add 2 drops to each side of your pillow to relieve insomnia

ORANGE

A CALMING AND RELAXING OIL

Botanical name *Citrus sinensis*

Plant part used Fruit peel.

Main benefits This oil has a refreshing and stimulating effect on the body whilst still leaving you relaxed. It rejuvenates skin. Excellent oil for calming children as well as for reducing colds and flu. Has antiseptic properties and is useful in the treatment of mouth ulcers.

Blending suggestions The light citrus aroma blends well with cypress, frankincense, lavender, neroli, petitgrain, rose and rosewood.

My comment Can be added to massage oil for muscle soreness.

Cautions This oil can cause irritation due to photosensitivity. Do not use when pregnant. Do not use within 72 hours of going in the sun.

POPULAR AROMATHERAPY OILS

(continued)

PATCHOULI
THE GENERAL TONIC OIL

Botanical name *Pogostemon cablin*

Plant part used Dried leaves.

Main benefits Useful in the treatment of eczema, acne, scalp and fungal infection of the skin. For anxiety and depression, patchouli helps keep one in touch with reality whilst encouraging spiritual wellbeing.

Blending suggestions The strong, exotic perfume of patchouli blends well with bergamot, clary sage, frankincense, geranium, ginger, lemongrass, neroli, rosewood, rose, sandalwood, and ylang ylang.

My comment Use in facial skin lotion to help reduce wrinkles.

Cautions Safe to use. Non-toxic.

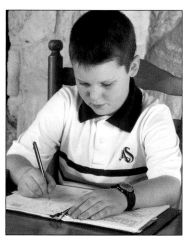

Helps concentration when studying

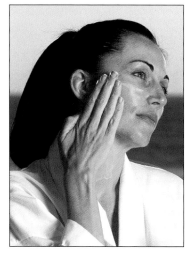

Use as a facial lotion to help reduce wrinkles

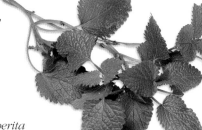

PEPPERMINT
THE SOOTHING DIGESTION OIL

Botanical name *Mentha piperita*

Plant part used Flowering tops and leaves.

Main benefits The cooling and refreshing effect on the body brings temporary relief from headaches, mental fatigue, toothache, sinusitis, travel sickness, sunburn, upset stomachs and hangovers.

Blending suggestions The strong, pungent, refreshing aroma of peppermint oil blends well with the citrus oils, basil, cypress, eucalyptus, marjoram, pine, rosemary and thyme.

My comment Improve your concentration by inhaling this oil when at work or studying.

Cautions Avoid during pregnancy. Use with care on sensitive skins – it can be an irritant due to high menthol content.

PETITGRAIN
THE NERVE OIL

Botanical name

Citrus auantium var. *amara*

Plant part used

Leaves from citrus trees.

Main benefits Petitgrain's
properties include being antidepressant,
deodorising and a sedative.

Blending suggestions Petitgrain's perfume is sweet and
a little sharp. It blends well with the other citrus oils as
well as clary sage, geranium and lavender.

My comment Use in your oil-warmer and inhale to
reduce depression and to clear a confused mind.

Cautions Non-toxic and safe to use at home.

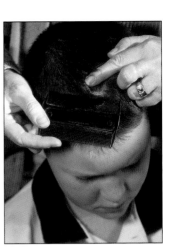
One of the best oils to treat head lice

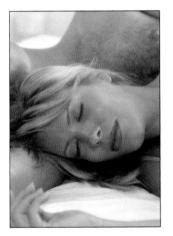
Petitgrain has a sedative effect

PINE
THE RESPIRATORY OIL

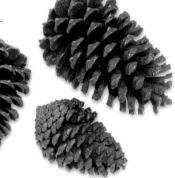

Botanical name

Pinus sylvestris

Plant part used

Needles, twigs
and cones.

Main benefits One of the best oils to treat head lice,
sores, cuts and scabies. Pine has a great effect on the
respiratory system and helps to loosen and remove
mucus. Useful in the treatment of bronchitis, coughs, sore
throats, colds, flu, asthma and for muscular aches and
pains, arthritis and rheumatism.

Blending suggestions The fresh, clean, camphor smell
blends well with cedarwood, cypress, eucalyptus,
lavender, sweet marjoram, peppermint, thyme and tea
tree.

My comment The perfect oil to benefit the respiratory
system. Use in oil-warmer, bath and massage oil.

Cautions It is non-toxic but it can be an irritant when
used in high doses on sensitive skins. Avoid massage oil
and bathing with pine for allergic skins.

POPULAR AROMATHERAPY OILS

(continued)

ROSE
THE BEAUTY OIL

Botanical name *Rosa damascene*

Plant part used Petals.

Main benefits Rose oil prevents and reduces scaring. It is a helpful oil for asthma and chronic bronchitis. The beautiful fragrance helps bring balance and harmony as well as stimulating and elevating the mind.

Blending suggestions Blends well with bergamot, chamomile, clary sage, geranium, jasmine, lavender, melissa, rosewood and ylang ylang.

My comment Use in facial treatments, ideal for all skin types. Use with calendula cream and chamomile for red and inflamed skin.

Cautions Non-toxic and safe to use.

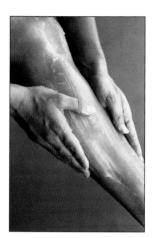

Relieves muscle soreness

ROSEMARY
THE OIL FOR PROTECTION

Botanical name

Rosmarinus officinalis

Plant part used

Flowering top and leaves.

Main benefits Rosemary is a powerful stimulant and has impressive healing properties, strengthening the nervous system, improving memory and restoring sense of smell. Rosemary can ease the pain of arthritis, gout, rheumatism, stiff and sore muscles. It is also used with success in treating asthma, colds, flu, bronchitis and coughs.

Blending suggestions The sharp penetrating perfume blends well with basil, cedarwood, all the citrus oils, lavender and peppermint.

My comment Use regularly as a hair-conditioning rinse. Use also to overcome mental fatigue and improve mental clarity and focus.

Cautions Avoid during pregnancy and if suffering from epilepsy.

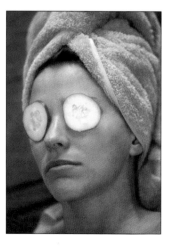

Great as a facial treatment

ROSEWOOD
A GENTLE BALANCING OIL

Botanical name

Aniba rosaeodora

Plant part used

Wood from the tropical evergreen tree.

Main benefits Rosewood is soothing, uplifting, refreshing and balancing. This oil is calming and relaxing for the emotions and gently sensual.

Blending suggestions The sweet, floral, wood aroma blends well with most other essential oils.

My comment Use in facial oils, creams and lotions, especially for dry and sensitive skins.

Cautions Non-toxic and safe to use.

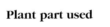

Rosewood makes a soothing body lotion

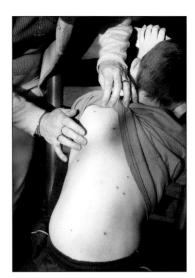

An effective treatment for blisters

TEA TREE
FIRST AID IN A BOTTLE

Botanical name

Melaleuca alternifolia

Plant part used

Leaves and twigs.

Main benefits Tea tree has many outstanding properties. It can be used to treat anything from blisters, boils, burns, rashes, gingivitis, mouth ulcers, burns, insect bites, nappy rash, ringworm to athlete's foot and thrush, infected wounds, coldsores, corns and warts.

Blending suggestions The resinous, slightly musty aroma of tea tree blends well with clary sage, cypress, eucalyptus, geranium, ginger, lavender, lemon, lemongrass, rosemary and thyme.

My comment Use as a gargle for throat and mouth infections.

Cautions Non-toxic and safe to use. Repeated neat application might induce sensitisation.

POPULAR AROMATHERAPY OILS

(continued)

THYME
NATURE'S ANTISEPTIC

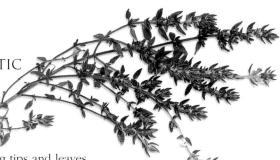

Botanical name

Thymus vulgaris

Plant part used Flowering tips and leaves.

Main benefits A powerful healer of skin; a stimulant to the immune and digestive systems; a disinfectant to the respiratory tract; a regulator of menstrual flow and a strengthener to the nervous system.

Blending suggestions The spicy, hot, nutmeg-like aroma blends well with bergamot, cedarwood, eucalyptus, lemon and rosemary.

My comment Use in the bath, as an inhalation on a tissue, or in a massage oil for relief from cold and flu symptoms.

Cautions Do not use on anyone with high blood pressure. Due to possible irritation factor use in moderation and only well diluted. Avoid during pregnancy.

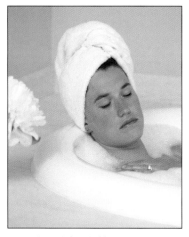

Use in the bath for relief from cold and flu symptoms

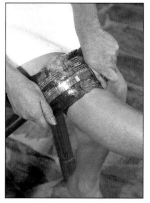

Use as a compress for arthritis pain

VETIVER
THE OIL OF TRANQUILLITY

Botanical name

Vetiveria zizanioides

Plant part used

Roots of wild grass.

Main benefits One of the best oils to use to strengthen the immune system. It is a deeply relaxing oil. Use in the bath to ease stress, lift depression, calm the nerves and for insomnia. Its antiseptic properties heal acne, cuts and infected wounds. Vetiver essential oil can be used during menopause to boost hormone secretions. During pregnancy, this oil improves the tone of slack and tired-looking skin.

Blending suggestions This dark brown, thick oil has an earthy aroma that blends well with clary sage, lavender, geranium, jasmine, patchouli and ylang ylang.

My comment Use in bath and compress for arthritis and rheumatism.

Cautions Non-toxic, non-irritant. Safe to use.

HOW TO USE ESSENTIAL OILS

Never use essential oils directly on the skin. There are a few exceptions which are detailed on page 68. For safe use, essential oils must always be diluted or diffused as follows:

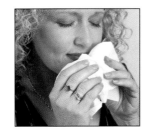

CARRIER OILS

In carrier oils for massage, friction rub, chest rub and pulse point application.

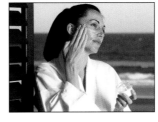

UNSCENTED BASE CREAMS

In unscented base creams for topical application in creams and lotions.

AIR

In the air through vaporisation, room and car fragrancing, candles, or in the sauna.

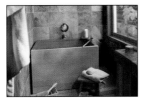

POWDER

In powder (rice flour or cornflour) to make foot and body powders.

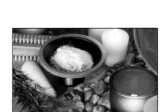

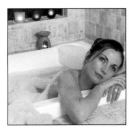

WATER

In water for baths, steam inhalation, as a compress, as a gargle/mouthwash, air fresheners, facial sprays and in the laundry.

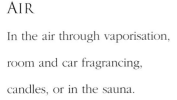

ALCOHOL

In alcohol to make eau de toilette and perfume.

NEAT

Neat, as in tissue inhalation, on your pillow, on logs of wood used on the fire, in drawers, cupboards and in bins.

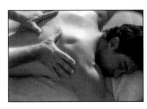

ESSENTIAL OILS DO NOT DISSOLVE IN WATER BUT DO DISSOLVE IN OIL.

When working with essential oils I recommend you use stainless steel, ceramic, glass or enamel containers and glass or stainless steel utensils. Do not use plastic bowls or utensils. For cloths or towels I recommend cotton and not synthetic fabrics.

Essential Oils In Carrier Oils

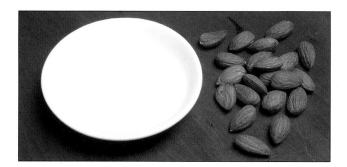

Carrier oils are used to dilute the essential oil in massage, friction rubs and pulse-point application. These carrier oils limit evaporation of the essential oil and speed the absorption into the skin. Oils can oxidise very easily. I recommend that you add 10% wheatgerm oil to your massage blend. Wheatgerm oil is rich in vitamins E and B, and in lecithin, and helps protect against oxidation. Oils that you buy in a supermarket are for cooking and might have been processed with a chemical agent or heat-treated. Carrier oils should be cold pressed and organic.

Following are the most popular vegetable carrier oils. These can be used 100% as your carrier oil.

SWEET ALMOND OIL

A fine, very pale yellow oil. Slow to become rancid. Rapidly absorbed; excellent for oily, sensitive skins. Recommended for body massage even in newborn babies. A useful source of Vitamin D.

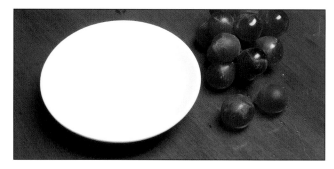

GRAPE SEED OIL

Very fine and clear, giving a satin-smooth finish without a greasy touch. Most often used as bath oil; needs to be dispersed well throughout the water.

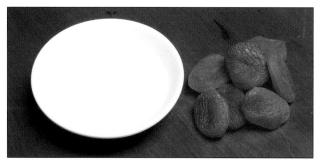

APRICOT KERNEL OIL

Pale yellow, rich in Vitamins E and A. Easily absorbed by the skin, nourishing and moisturising, it is suitable for facial treatments. Especially suitable for sensitive and inflamed dry skin.

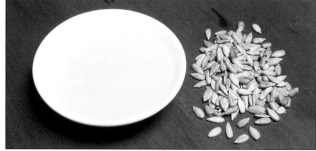

SUNFLOWER OIL

Pale yellow. Contains proteins, minerals and Vitamin F (an essential fatty acid). It has an excellent shelf life.

Other popular vegetable carrier oils that you can include 10% in your massage blend are:

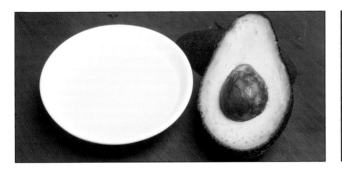

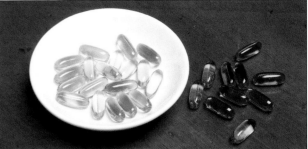

AVOCADO OIL

Rich, nourishing and compatible with the skin's own sebum. High in Vitamins A, C and E, it aids regeneration of scarred skin. Recommended for facial and body treatments; although thick, it leaves the skin feeling smooth and silky. Useful in treating dry and mature skin as well as nappy rash and eczema.

EVENING PRIMROSE OIL

Excellent, pale-yellow carrier oil, rich in fatty acids, particularly gamma linolenic acid (GLA). This acid affects much enzyme activity in the body. Effective in the treatment of eczema, rheumatoid arthritis, psoriasis, premenstrual syndrome and weight reduction when used as a massage oil.

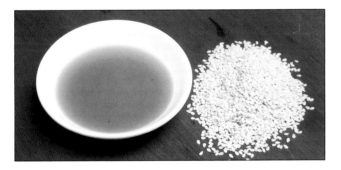

SESAME OIL

Dark-yellow carrier oil, rich in Vitamin A, E, minerals, protein and lecithin. Keeps well. Excellent for treating eczema and psoriasis.
A powerful anti-oxidant. It is used extensively in Ayurvedic treatments.

Other popular carrier oils:

JOJOBA OIL

The most luxurious of all the carrier oils. It is in fact a wax pressed from the bean of the plant. It does not go rancid. Light and rich in vitamin E. Gives a satin-smooth finish and feel to the skin. Offers an ideal base for perfume and luxurious face-moisturising oil. Useful in treating acne, eczema, psoriasis and inflamed skin.

WHEAT GERM OIL

Rich, nourishing, fine healing oil, yellow–orange in colour. It contains proteins, minerals and Vitamin E and is perfect for anti-stretchmark blends.

AROMATHERAPY MASSAGE

PREPARING FOR A MASSAGE

PREPARE YOURSELF

- Be sure your nails are short and clean

- Wear comfortable clothes

- Remove all jewellery

- Wash hands before each massage

- Drink a full glass of filtered or spring water

MAKE SURE YOU HAVE EVERYTHING TO HAND SO THERE ARE NO INTERRUPTIONS

- A futon, a yoga mat or a large spongy mat on the floor is fine

- A small table close at hand

- Carrier oil and pure essential oil mix in a bowl

- Basin of boiling water to warm small bowl of mixed oil

- Enough towels – bath sheets and smaller towels

- Eye bag

- Box of tissues

- Three pillows

- A head rest

- Heater to warm the towels

- An essential oil-warmer burning with relaxing essential oils

- Have a hot water bottle handy for under the feet

- Have a glass of water to offer the person you are massaging

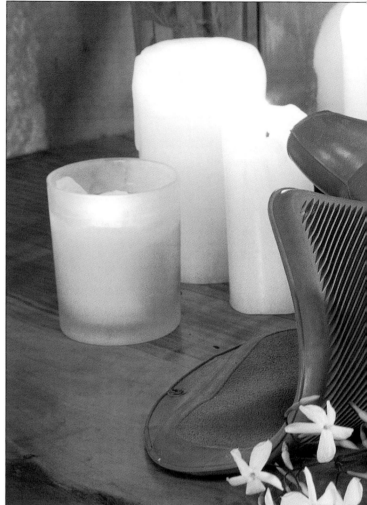

SET THE MOOD FOR A SNUG, COMFORTABLE AND RELAXED ENVIRONMENT

- Make sure there is no draught

- In winter heat the room

- Ensure dim lighting – no bright overhead lights

- Play soft, soothing music

- Unplug the phones or put on message bank and switch off mobile phones.

- Put note on door – DO NOT DISTURB

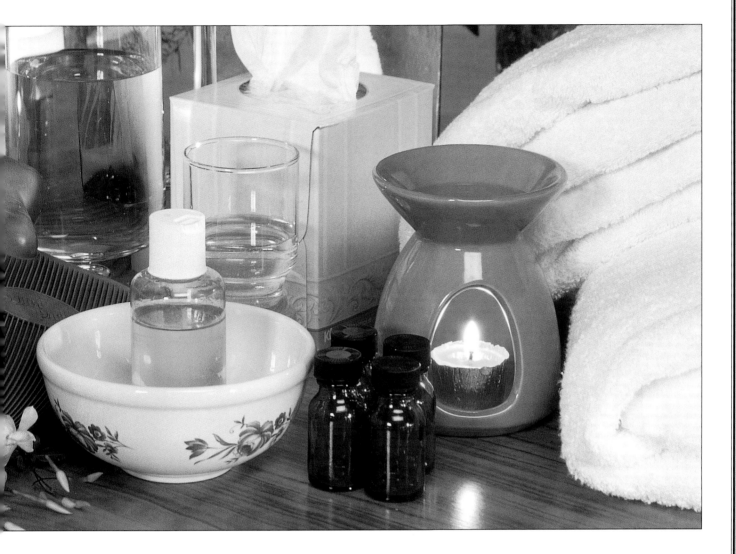

MENTAL PREPARATION

As you prepare the room, light the candle burner and add the oils to clear any negative energy that might be in the area. Take a deep breath, relax for a few minutes, concentrate on your breathing. As you breathe in visualise taking in heaps of clean oxygenated air. As you breathe out visualise your muscles relaxing as you expel the carbon dioxide with all your 'stuff' of the day. Visualise it leaving your body and being dispelled by the burning light of the candle. Visualise putting any pressing problems you have into a drawer and closing it, leaving your mind relaxed and present in the moment for the massage.

AROMATHERAPY MASSAGE SEQUENCE

INTRODUCTION

There are various different strokes and techniques used in massage. In this sequence you will learn opening and closing techniques, effleurage, kneading, stroking thumbs/finger circles, sweeping, fanning, circling movements, the figure of 8, percussion, stretching, the corkscrew, finger press and pinching.

Begin by connecting with your subject and becoming fully aware of your breathing . This is done with your subject fully covered with towels.

Position yourself at your subject's side. With your hands above their body as you clear your thoughts, relax, breathe, and begin to feel the energy flowing into your hands as you breathe in. Place one hand at the base of the spine and the other at the top of the spine. Rest for a moment. Note any sensations or impressions.

Ask your subject to breathe in and out three times using deep abdominal breathing. This helps your subject to let go and slow their mind and body.

Without losing contact with the body, position yourself at the subject's head and gently rest your fingers on their hairline as they breathe in. Ask them to breathe in again and to visualise any 'stuff' coming up for them that they need to let go of. As they breathe out, drag your fingers like a rake through their hair and flick off at the end of their hair. Rake through their hair with your fingers three times. You are now ready to begin the full body massage.

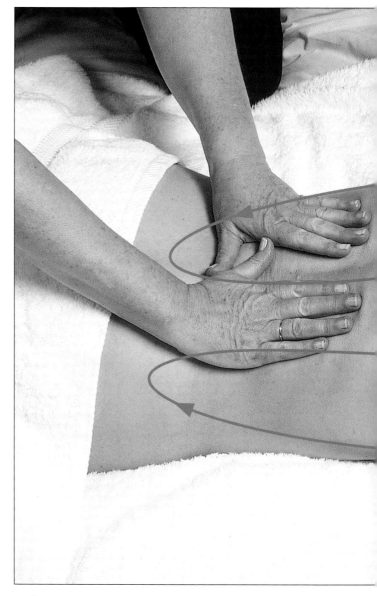

1. Effleurage

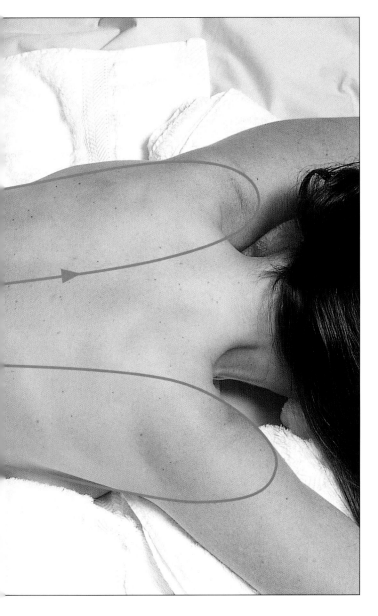

BACK AND BUTTOCKS

Effleurage is a gentle, fan-like stroke used at the beginning of the massage. It helps to spread the oil over the skin, relaxing the surface of the skin. This stroke uses the palm of the hand, with fingers and wrists relaxed. The movements feel smooth and rhythmic. Effleurage can be done at any point through the massage to connect different strokes.

EFFLEURAGE

1. Gently fold the towel down the back to the middle of the buttocks. Pour just enough oil into your palms, rub hands together, position yourself at the lower back, facing the body. Slowly slide both hands up the spine to the neck. Fan both hands over each shoulder, cupping and embracing the upper arm as you slide your hands to the underarm position, then slowly slide lightly down the sides of the body to the starting position. Repeat rhythmically several times till the oil is well spread. The slow rhythmic movement of this stroke is deeply relaxing.

AROMATHERAPY MASSAGE SEQUENCE

(continued)

KNEADING

This is a medium-pressure stroke. It is used after the muscles have been relaxed and oil has been spread over the skin. This technique is like kneading dough. You will be working more deeply to further relax the muscles, release general tension and increase circulation. Place hands flat, fingers together with thumbs stretched out wide. Using your thumb to push in, squeeze and pinch the flesh towards the fingers, scooping up the skin. The hands work alternately, pressing and squeezing the muscles in a rolling movement. Kneading speeds up blood and lymph flow.

2. Position yourself square to the body. Lean across and press into the opposite buttock with your thumbs spread wide as they roll towards the fingers of the same hand. Work your hands in a rhythmic movement, alternately up the side, from the sacrum, across over hip joint, up the side of the ribs in a rhythmic movement, working upwards toward the shoulder. This can be a very tense and painful area so work sensitively. Work in two rows, buttock to shoulder, on both sides of the spine.

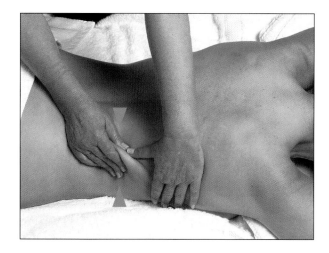

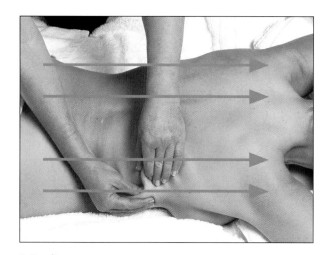

2. Kneading

THUMB CIRCLES

Make small rhythmic circles with your thumb or fingertips. As you circle, the pressure continues downwards. Always check your pressure is causing no discomfort or pain. When you come across a knot, gently work through it, increasing pressure as it releases. To relax a muscle, begin pressure, gently increasing it when you feel a response. Continue circling the area a few times and then move on, so as not to cause resistance or irritation.

3. Position yourself at your subject's lower back. Work with both thumbs alongside each other at the same time. Perform small continuous circles from the sacrum to the base of the skull three times on each side of the spine.

Cautions Do not work *on* the spine – work on either side of the vertebrae.

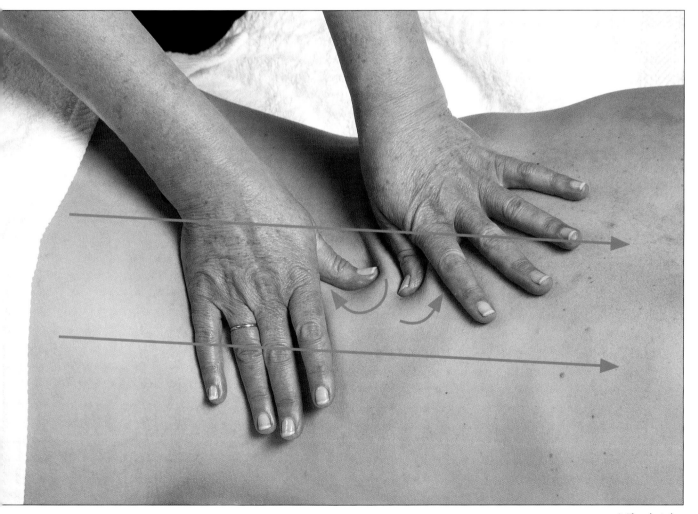

3. Thumb circles

AROMATHERAPY MASSAGE SEQUENCE

(continued)

STROKING

This is the simplest movement, with palms down and hands flat (on large areas) and curved (around small areas). It is one of the gentle light-pressure techniques. You can do it with your fingers only, or you can cat stroke: one hand follows the other and curves so only the fingertips touch at the end of the stroke. It can be performed at the end of massage sequences. Stroking is pleasurable and connects sensations to the area that has just been massaged. It draws attention to that part of the body, relaxing, revitalising and stimulating the skin. When performed slowly, it has a calming and soothing effect. When performed with fast rapid strokes it is invigorating.

4. Position yourself square to the body with flat hands, straight fingers, stroke away from you from the middle of the spine to the side of the body. Start at the shoulder and finish at the hips and back again. Repeat on the other side of spine, stroking towards you. Begin at the shoulder. Alternatively, position yourself at the head, reach to the lower back, place one hand on the sacrum and cat stroke with alternating hands all the way up the spine to the skull. Repeat three times.

SWEEPING

This is a light to medium stroke using the palm and fingers held flat. It is used after squeezing the muscles to relax, stretch and open them out. The strokes are worked in quick succession, one hand after the other, with pressure away from the spine when working the back and hip area.

5. Position yourself at the hip and lightly place your hands on the far side of the hip and buttock. Sweep hands alternately one after the other in a downward movement away from you towards the side of the body. Repeat the stroke, moving slowly toward the shoulder with each sweep. Repeat from buttock to shoulder again. Repeat on the other side.

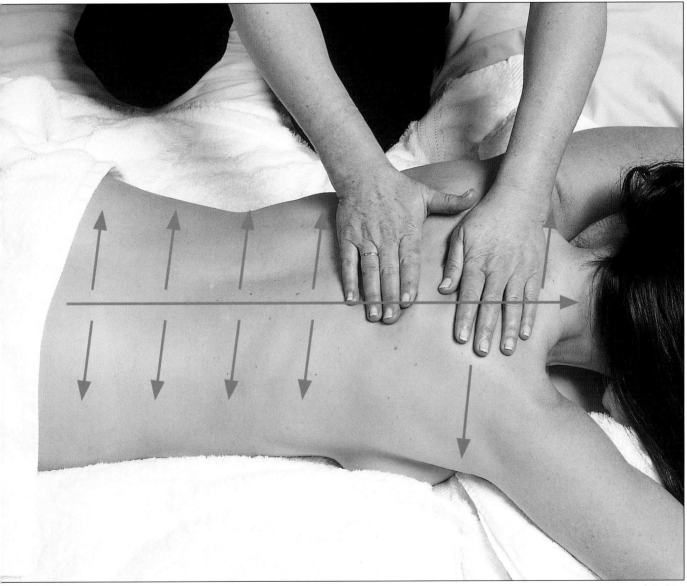

4. Stroking

AROMATHERAPY MASSAGE SEQUENCE

(continued)

FANNING

Is a light to medium stroke performed with flat hands and straight fingers. Palms of your hands should pivot as fingers fan over the body.

6. Position yourself at the side of your subject with flat hands placed on the shoulder. The first stroke applies firm downward pressure. You lighten the pressure as you fan over the shoulder and continue with alternating hands down the spine, fanning outward to the side and moving downward to the hip. Repeat on the other side.

CIRCLING OVER BUTTOCKS

Here your hands are in the same position as for stroking, only they move in circles. You place one hand on the other, palms down and make one single circle. This stroke is very comforting and relaxing; it is perfect for a subject who is upset.

7. Position yourself at the hip area. Place both hands gently and flat, one on top of the other, in the middle of the opposite buttock. Use gentle pressure in slow, rhythmic circles several times.

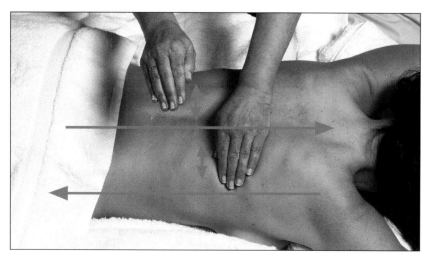

8a. Cupping

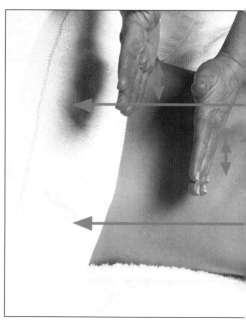

8b. Hacking

PERCUSSION

This is a series of three strokes – cupping, hacking and pummeling. Work from the buttocks to the shoulder and back, one hand following the other in rapid succession. The movements are brisk with firm pressure. Work up one side and down the other.

8a. Cupping: Cup your hand forming a vacuum in the palm of your hand, fingers straight and thumb pulled tight in. As you cup the skin with one hand flick off immediately, followed by the other hand doing the same.

8b. Hacking: Hold hands straight with palms facing. Hack the skin with the sides of your hands, one hand following the other. As your hand touches the skin bounce off immediately.

8c. Pummeling: Form an open fist closing the top with your thumb. Pummel the skin briskly, bouncing off on contact, alternating each hand in rhythmic succession.

Caution: Take care not to strike delicate areas – work on muscles either side of spine – See the muscle chart, page 9.

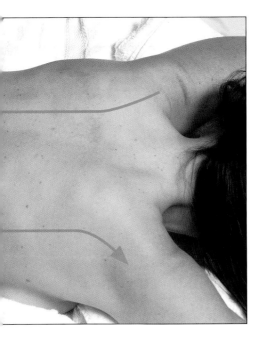

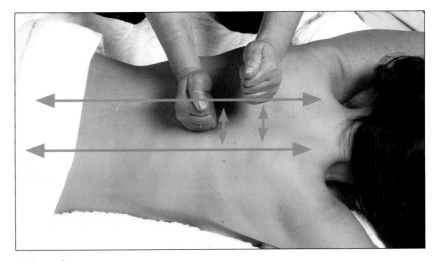

8c. Pummeling

AROMATHERAPY MASSAGE SEQUENCE

(continued)

FIGURE OF 8

The number 8 represents infinity. It is considered the most active spiritual number, the number of wisdom, being intuition expressed through loving action. This technique is similar to circling but in a figure of 8, with both hands working at the same time in opposite directions. The pressure is medium to firm. It is used near the end of massaging a body part, when the area is warm and relaxed. Use varying pressure during the stroke. As you go over bony parts, the pressure is light while over the muscle you can increase the pressure.

9. Position yourself at one side of your subject, starting with one hand on either side of the buttock.
Move the hands with firm pressure as you circle in opposite directions and cross at the sacrum. Move smoothly up the back, repeating three figures of 8 in each position, till you finish with a set of figure of 8 across the shoulders.

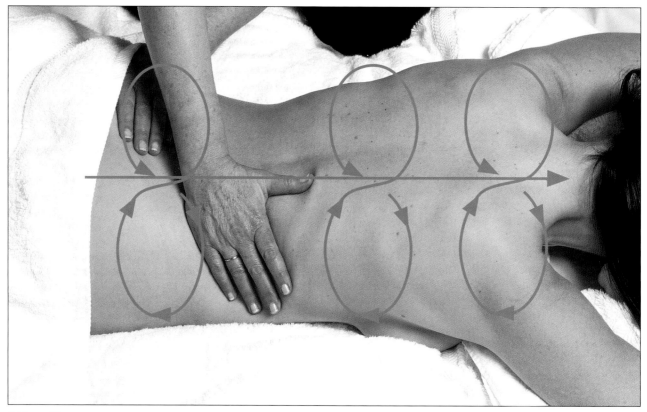

9. Figure of 8

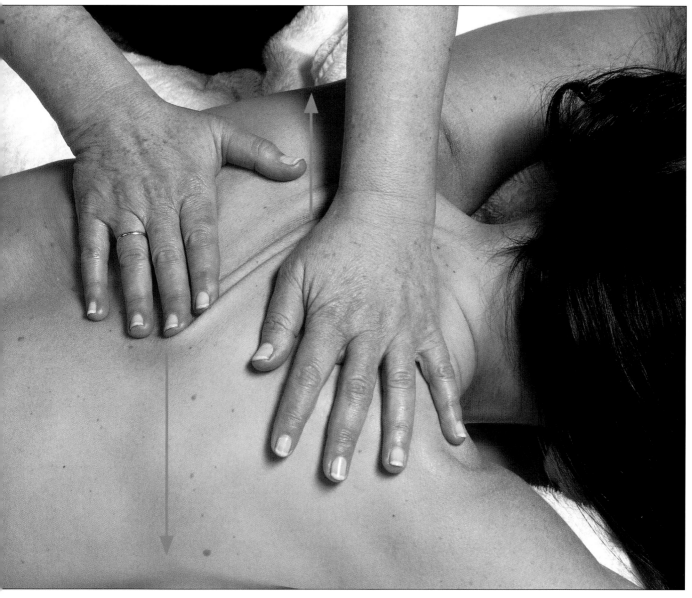

WRINGING

This stroke is done criss-crossing from side to side firmly.

This creates warm friction on muscle fibre.

10. Work from hips to shoulder blade and back again three times. For complete relaxation work slowly. For an invigorating effect speed up the tempo. Continuously stroke your hands in opposite directions as you wring the entire back region.

AROMATHERAPY MASSAGE SEQUENCE

(continued)

STRETCHING

This stroke has a firm, very slow, downward pressure of the hands, palms flat (abdomen, arms and legs), palms facing each other (back), whilst sliding hands apart diagonally in opposite directions. You can also turn them in opposite directions to twist and wring as you stretch. On the abdomen, the pressure should be medium not firm. This stroke gives the body a sense of opening out and not being held in.

11. Face your subject and position yourself at their waist. Bring your palms together, then place them in the middle of the back on the spine. Place pressure on the muscles on either side of the spine but not on the vertebrae. Slowly, very slowly with firm pressure, draw the hands apart feeling the muscle move beneath the side edge of your hands. If you do not feel it, you are moving too fast. Slide in opposite directions, one hand to the sacrum the other to the top of the neck. Hold the finish for a few seconds with firm pressure. Lift and place hands quickly once again in the middle of the back on the spine, and slide one hand to the hip the other to the shoulder. Repeat, moving the hands to the opposite hip and shoulder.

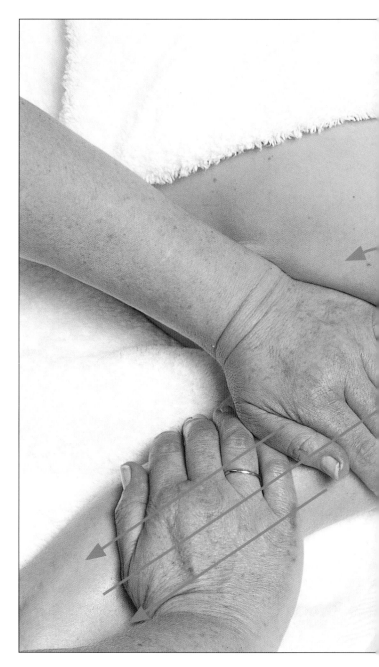

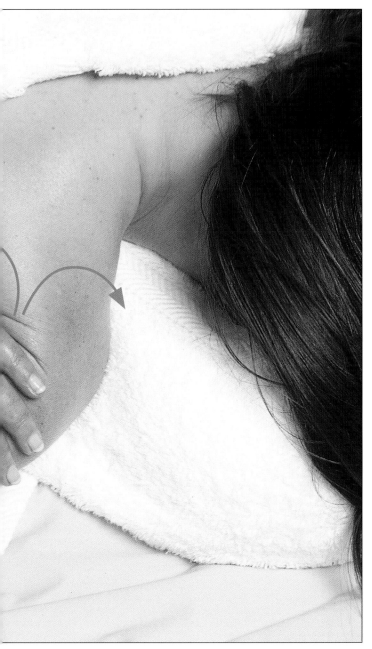

1. Effleurage of the arms

TO FINISH THE BACK AND BUTTOCKS

Complete three, rhythmic effleurage strokes. The first medium pressure, the second light pressure and slowing in pace, the last featherlight and very slow.

Draping – bring the towel back and cover the body completely. Rest one hand on the towel at the top of the spine and the other hand at the base of the spine as you connect with your subject. Rest for a few seconds. You are now ready to start the arms. Fold corner of towel exposing entire arm and shoulder area.

AROMATHERAPY MASSAGE SEQUENCE

(continued)

ARMS

1. Uncover one arm. Effleurage the arm from hand to shoulder three times as you apply oil.

2. Knead upper arm with a sliding movement, applying pressure with the thumbs. Repeat three times on the inside and three times on the outside. Supporting the arm, complete three hand circles on the elbow with a flat palm and pressure on the inside of the elbow. Knead the lower arm three times with pressure on the inside of wrists.

3. Do knuckle circles into the palm of the hand.

CORKSCREW OFF EACH FINGER

This is a gentle but firm sliding, twisting and pulling stroke. It can be done on fingers and toes.

4. Hold the subject's hand at the wrist, with your other hand. Curl all four fingers of your hand around each finger one at a time. Twist gently as you slide off each finger starting with the thumb. Twist off each finger pulling gently as you slide off. Finish with the little finger.

5. Three effleurage strokes up the arm to finish. Firm, lighter and fairy lightness to finish. Repeat all five steps on the other arm.

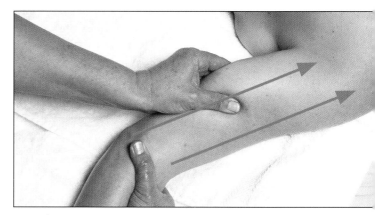
2. Knead upper arm

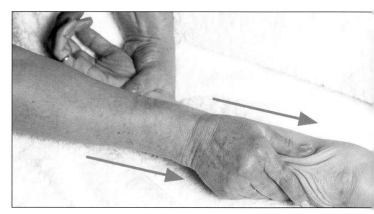
2. Knead lower arm

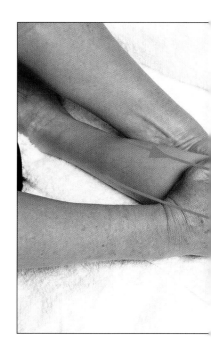

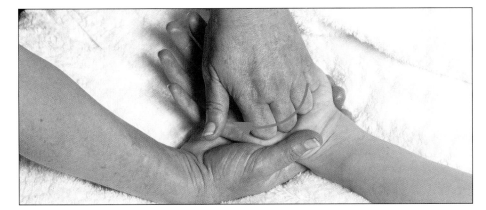

3. Knuckle circling

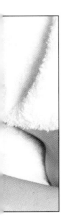

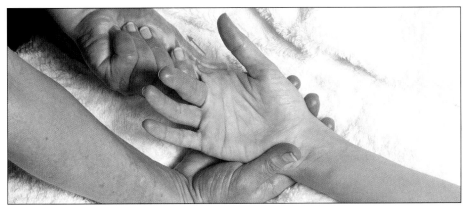

4. Corkscrew off each finger

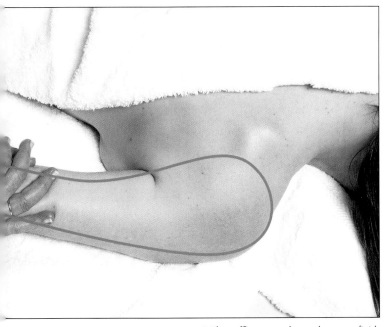

5. Three effleurage strokes up the arm to finish

To complete massaging this side of the body: place one hand on the neck and the other at the base of the spine. Hold for a few seconds and visualise your subject completely relaxed. Lift the towel to screen your face and ask your subject to turn over. For comfort, place a pillow under the knees. Offer your subject an eye pad to assist relaxation. Place support under the neck if necessary. Ask if they are warm enough. You are now ready to massage the front of the body.

AROMATHERAPY MASSAGE SEQUENCE

(continued)

FRONT AND BACK OF LEGS

1. Effleurage the full front of the leg three times as you apply oil. First on the lower leg, then either side of the knee, then the upper leg.

2. Knead the upper front leg then the lower front leg. Three times each in three lines. Use very light sliding pressure on shin bone.

3. Run finger circles around each side of the ankle. This is the same as the thumb circle but using one, two or three fingers. Complete three circles, working both hands on either side of the ankle at the same time.

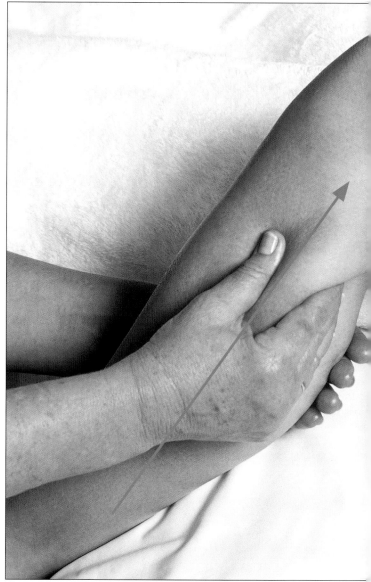

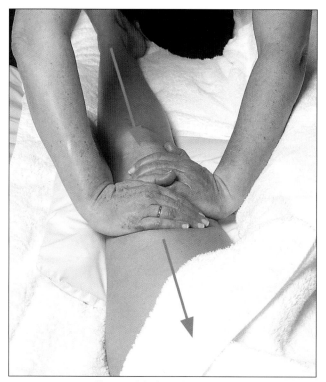

1. Effleurage of the front of the leg three times as you apply oil

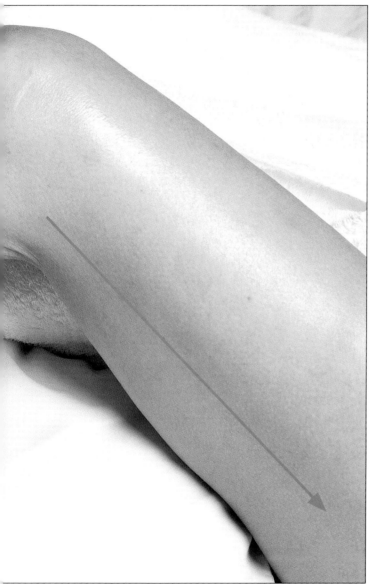

5. Knead the back of the leg

4. Gently slide one hand under the knee, the other hand on ankle. Push ankle whilst lifting the knee into a 45° angle and secure foot with corner of towel. Use more oil if necessary using effleurage stroke.

5. First knead the calf and through the thigh. Work both sides of the leg three times each, first on the lower leg and then on the upper leg.

AROMATHERAPY MASSAGE SEQUENCE

(continued)

KNEES, ANKLES, FEET

6. Complete circles around the knee with palm and finger. Both hands following each other.

7. Do finger circles around each side of the ankle. Hold the ankle between your wrists and gently rock from side to side three times.

8. Foot stretch. Slide both hands around the foot and stretch the top of the foot with thumbs facing up. Slide firmly to the outside of the foot whilst fingers are exerting pressure into the solar plexus. Repeat three times.

9. Toe circles. Hold each toe one at a time, gently circle clockwise then anticlockwise and corkscrew off. Move to the next toe till all toes are massaged.

10. Foot twist. Place one hand on the inside of the foot and your other hand on the outside of the foot. Using the heels of the hand pull the outside of their foot towards you with one hand as you push the inside of the foot away from you and visa versa. Work along the edges of the foot from the heels to the toes and back again three times. This technique loosens the lower back, upper back and shoulders.

To finish, effleurage from toe to thigh three times. The first time apply medium pressure, the second time light pressure and slowing in pace, the last time feather-light and very slowly. Hold both your hands still on the foot for a few seconds. Visualise all tension leaving the entire body. Cover and repeat on the other leg.
Repeat step 1 - 10 on the other leg.

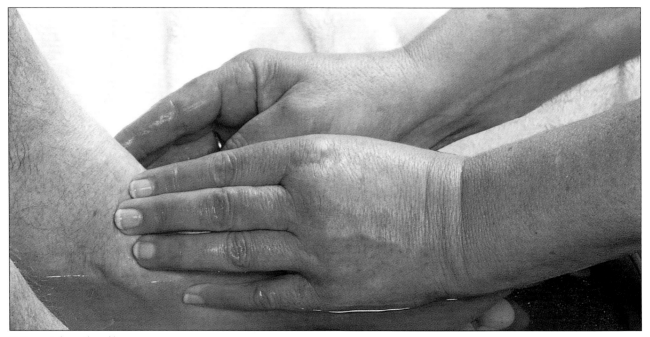

7. Finger circles on the ankle

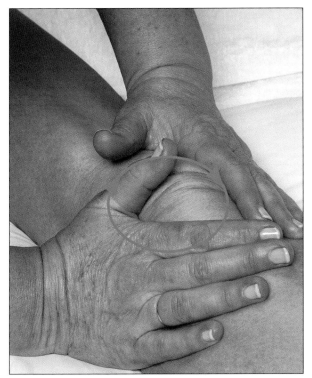

6. Hand circles

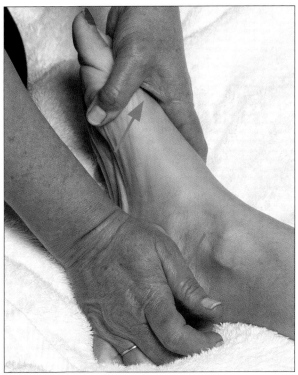

8. Foot stretch

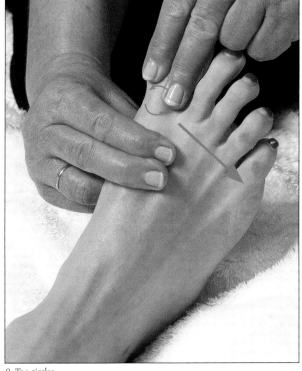

9. Toe circles

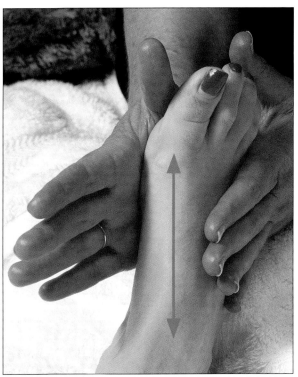

10. Foot twist

AROMATHERAPY MASSAGE SEQUENCE

(continued)

ABDOMEN

Drape the chest with a towel (for women). Fold a towel in half lengthwise and place half over one shoulder, make a 'V' over the breast area and fold the other half over the other shoulder. Pull the towel covering the breast area down to hips whilst securing the 'V' towel in place. Position yourself at the right side of your subject.

1. Effleurage the abdomen in clockwise circles.

Apply the oil with flat hands. Starting in a small circle, very gently apply pressure and make larger and larger circles. Repeat several times. This is a very calming technique.

2. Place hands, palms flat, on the abdomen below the navel. Rest there for a few seconds, tuning into your subject's breathing. As your subject breathes out, apply gentle pressure with the flat of your hands. Draw your

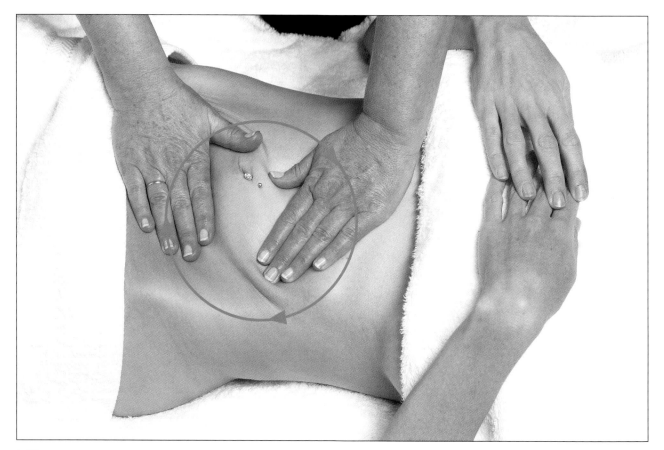

1. Effleurage

hands apart, sliding towards the hips. Stretch outwards. Do not dig in. Gently tuck hands under the hips, lift slightly and rock gently from side to side. Repeat three times. Should your subject have a navel ring slightly cup your hands. Rest the hands there for the count of three as you tune in. Then, very slowly, move both hands in slow, rhythmic and continuous circles, starting with a very small circle over the navel. Repeat these circles, moving clockwise, making larger circles until you are covering the entire tummy area. Do many large circles before you start to go smaller and finish in the starting position. Hold that position for the count of 20.

3. To finish, place the right hand flat on solar plexus (between ribs). With very gentle pressure, circle five times very slowly in a clockwise direction, hold for a few seconds and remove. Replace drape. Fold both top ends of the 'V' back over chest exposing both shoulders, top of the chest and neck area.

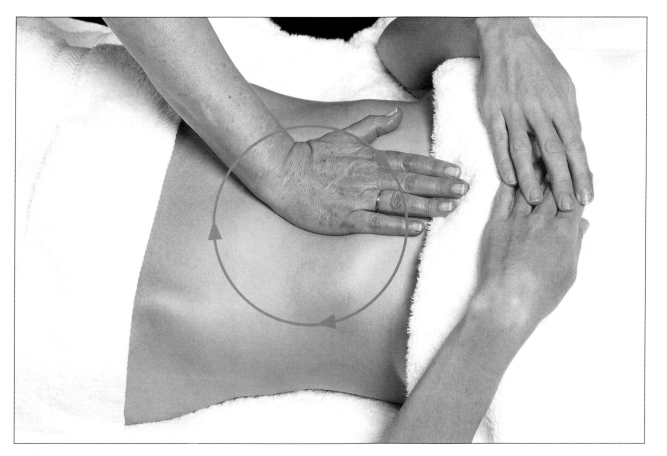

3. Solar Plexus

AROMATHERAPY MASSAGE SEQUENCE

(continued)

CHEST, NECK AND SHOULDERS

1. Stand at your subject's head. Effleurage the entire area with oil, starting with both hands in the middle of the chest; slide over shoulders, behind the neck and slowly up the back of the neck, taking in the ears with your fingers and then sliding gently off under the head and the hair. Repeat three times slowly and rhythmically.

2. Finger press. Place both hands in the middle of the chest, fingers resting between the ribs. Press slowly and evenly between the top ribs, starting in the centre and moving outwards in three position. Apply firm pressure and hold for a few seconds. Slide along between ribs and press again. Repeat three times. Be careful not to put pressure on breast tissue. This step stimulates the neurolymphatic reflex points. Repeat with thumbs only, in two positions at the armpit.

3. Shoulder press. With one hand on left shoulder and one on the right gently press right shoulder down; then press left shoulder, then together. Repeat three times. Always work rhythmically.

4. Shoulder effleurage with flat hands. Work both hands together from shoulder to shoulder and back again three times.

5. Effleurage the neck starting in the middle of the chest. Move outwards to the shoulders and end with both hands underneath the neck with your fingers at either side of the spine. Make small finger circles inward to the neck and repeat three times. Support the head with one hand and gently turn the head to the left. Effleurage from the shoulder up the back of the neck to hairline. Firmly massage scalp from base of skull to top of head with fingers spread wide. Move the scalp not the hair. Supporting the head, gently turn to other side and repeat. This stimulating action on the scalp improves circulation, increases blood flow, nourishes the hair follicles and stimulates nerve endings. You are now ready to start massaging the face.

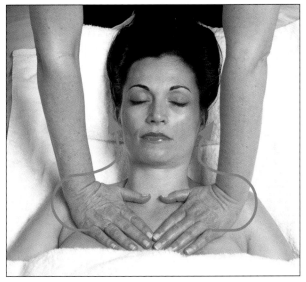

1. Effleurage starting on chest

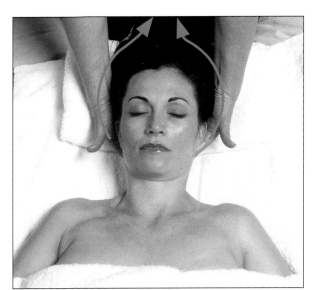

1. Effleurage complete by sliding under head and off hair

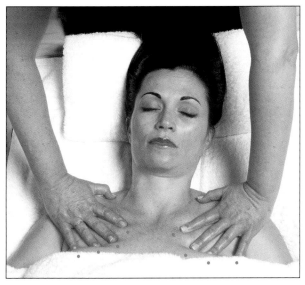

2. Finger press

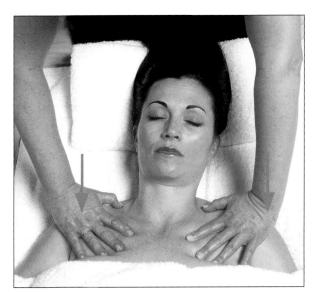
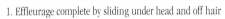

3. Shoulder press

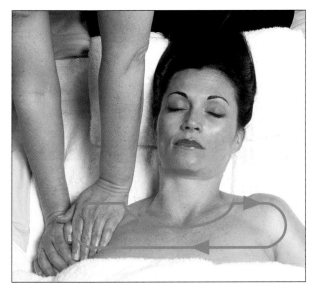

4. Shoulder effleurage

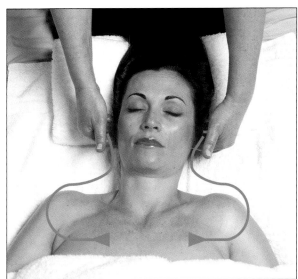

5. Final effleurage and scalp massage

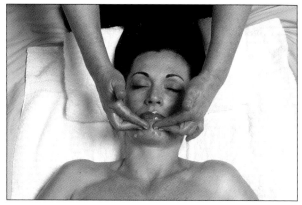
4. Lower lip

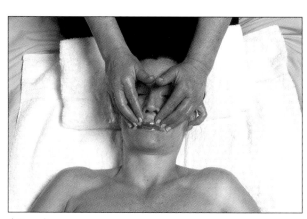
4. Upper lip

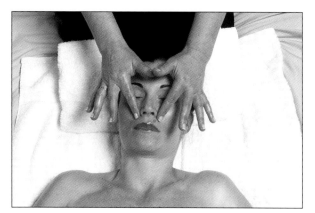
5. Sinus finger press

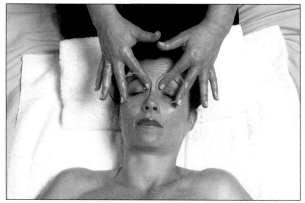
6. Eye circles

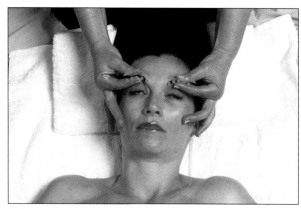
7. Eyebrow pinch

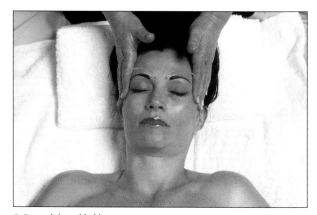
8. Press, slide and hold

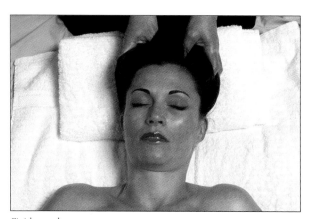
Finish – scalp massage

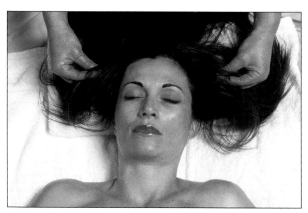
Finish – rake the hair

AROMATHERAPY MASSAGE SEQUENCE

(continued)

FACE

1. Using the palms of the hand, effleurage the entire face with oil, with both hands mirroring each other. Work gentle strokes with fingertips from forehead to chin, over nose and with care around the eyes.

2. Place the heel of your hands on the forehead. Stroke rhythmically outwards towards the temples. Hold and release. Repeat three times.

3. Massage the chin. Use sideways movements from the middle of the chin, along the jaw bone to under the ears with fingers underneath and thumbs working in circles. Pat gently under jaw line with the ring and middle fingers in a bouncing percussion movement.

4. Gently press five times below the lower lip using your middle three finger pads. Repeat on the upper lip. This helps to relax the jaw.

5. Gently press five times on acupressure point at the side of nose using your pointer finger pads. This is used to relieve sinus problems.

6. With your pointer finger, draw up from the base of the nose to under the eyebrow. Apply gentle finger press three times then glide three times along the eyebrow circle over the temple and back under the eyes to the nose. This is amazingly relaxing, relieving all anxiety and tension.

7. Using your thumb and forefinger gently pinch firmly five times along the eyebrow. This technique relieves eyestrain and sinus congestion. Repeat three times.

8. Place your thumbs together on the forehead above the brows. Start at the third eye (between the eyebrows). Press lightly downwards, hold, release. Then stroke out across the forehead to the temples with pads and fingers and hold. Repeat this press, slide and hold stroke three times. The slower and more even the pressure, the more effective the stroke. The movement should be delicate as if drawing tension away from the centre of the face **To finish.** Massage the scalp all over with firm finger circles. Move the scalp. Do not slide on the hair. Now, rake the head in three lines starting at the hairline – very slowly with stiff, rake-like fingers glide from hairline all the way along the scalp and off the ends of the hair, flicking off as you finish. This cleansing action draws negative energy from the head and the hair. Complete the massage with a final effleurage over the chest, shoulders, up the back of the neck, include the ears, and off the hair. Repeat three times, getting slower and lighter each time. Finish with your thumbs gently positioned on the crown of the head, gently moving on the spot up and down for several moves. Cover your subject. Replace the eye bag. End the treatment by placing the palms of your hands on the soles of their feet for at least 10 seconds. This re-balances the flow of energy. Leave your subject for five minutes to allow the energy to settle. Wash your hands. Come back with a glass of water. Ask them to keep their eyes closed and take a deep breath in as you gently spritz their face. Repeat three times.

ESSENTIAL OILS IN CARRIER OILS

(continued)

PULSE POINT MASSAGE

Add one drop of lavender pure essential oil to 1 ml carrier oil for headache relief.

Blend oil, then use your pointer and middle finger on each pulse-point to massage into the four pulse points – at wrist, upper arm, on the neck at jugular vein, and at the temples.

Technique: apply pressure on point, hold for the count of three. Complete three small circles clockwise and three circles anticlockwise, then hold for the count of three. Move to the next pulse point. It is important to drink one glass of water before you start and one glass of water when you are finished. Drink 2 litres of water over the next 24 hours. Try to maintain this level of water every day. This is an easy, quick way to enable essential oils to enter the bloodstream and can be used successfully to treat problems such as headaches, insomnia, lack of concentration and cold and flu.

FRICTION RUB MASSAGE

Place a small amount of the blended oil in the palm of your hand and rub both hands together fast until they warm up. Take three deep breaths of the oil to assist sleep. You can friction rub children's feet to calm them at sleep time.

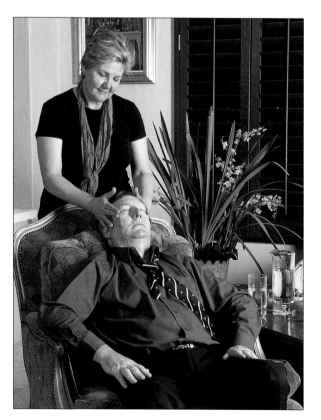

Pulse point massage on temples

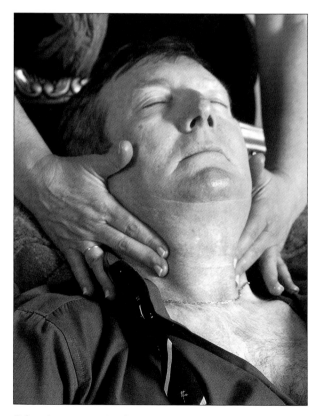

Pulse point massage on jugular vein

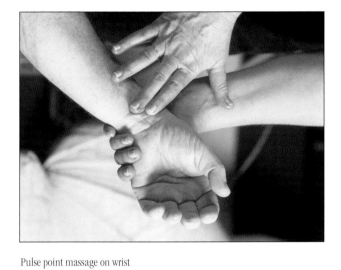

Pulse point massage on wrist

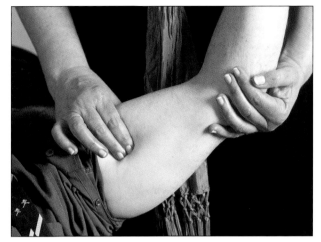

Pulse point massage on upper arm

Friction rub or massage children's feet to help sleep (1 drop of lavender pure essential oil in 2 teaspoons of carrier oil)

ESSENTIAL OILS IN THE AIR

OIL WARMERS

As essential oils are gently heated in the warmer, the highly volatile oils turn into vapours, and you receive the therapeutic effect by breathing them in the air. One of the most common ways of warming essential oils is to use an electric essential oil warmer.

ELECTRIC OIL WARMER

These are safer than candle warmers, as there is no fire threat with the electric warmer. Place 6–8 drops of pure essential oil in the ceramic indentation and switch on. No water is required in the bowl. To clean the surface, wipe with a clean cloth dipped in pure eucalyptus oil.

CANDLE OIL WARMER

This warmer uses a tea candle and can be a fire hazard. Although they look romantic, you can never be sure of the quality of the candles. Beeswax candles are the best. Add sufficient water to the dish, add 6–8 drops of essential oil and light the candle. Be sure to keep a check on the water level.

CAR FRESHENERS

Sprinkle a few drops on a tissue/cottonwool ball and place it in the air vent. Basil, peppermint, lemon and eucalyptus will help keep you alert on a long trip and will also freshen stale air.

CANDLES

Add 2 drops of your chosen essential oil to the melted wax of a candle that has been burning for a short while.

The warmth quickly diffuses the aroma into the air. Some essential oils are flammable so blow the candle out when you add the oil and relight the candle with care.

IN A SAUCER

If you do not have an oil warmer, you can put a little water and 6 drops of essential oil in a ceramic/glass saucer, and place it near or just in front of the room heater. The subtle aroma will pervade the air. Alternatively, place a dish of boiling water in a sunny window or in front of the fire and add a few drops of essential oil.

LIGHT BULB RING

This is a circular ring (made of absorbent material) with a hole to fit over a light bulb. Add 3–8 drops of essential oil to the ring and fit over a light bulb.

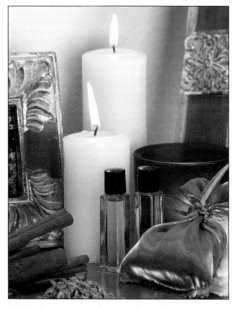

Diffuse the aroma into the air with candles

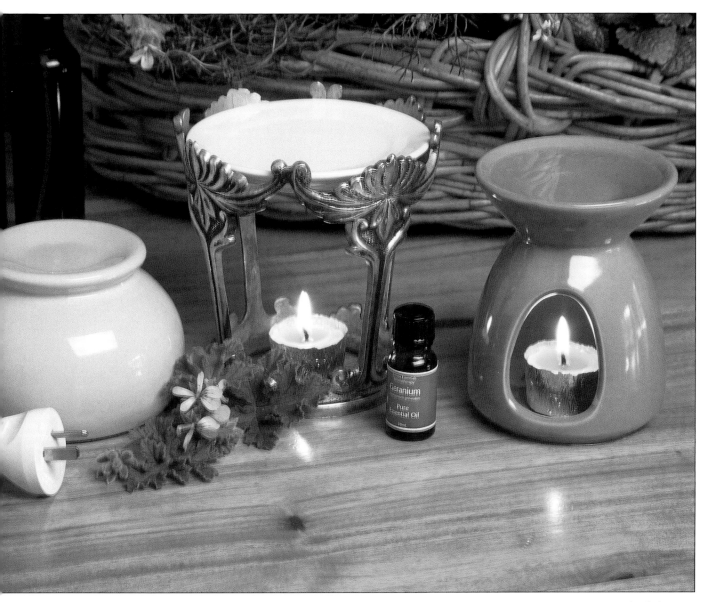

Various styles of oil warmer

ESSENTIAL OILS IN WATER

I hope I can convince you to introduce one of these pampering treats into your health and wellbeing regime. A hand or foot bath is one of the most effective ways to relieve stress and the next best thing to having an aromatherapy massage. For all water treatments be aware of temperature.

BATH TIME

A bath reduces tension and anxiety, calms the nervous system, enhances the removal of waste from the body, clears heat, fever and inflammation, improves circulation of blood and lymph and reduces pain.

Place 6–8 drops of essential oil in 1 tablespoon carrier oil and add to your full bath. Hop in, swirl the water around and enjoy. Essential oils have a very subtle effect. Do not expect to feel the effect as soon as you lie back – the effect will be felt in the hours that follow.

If you do not have any carrier oil, take a 'Cleopatra' bath.

Queen Cleopatra bathed in ass's milk.

The high-fat content of ass's milk dispersed and diluted the exotic Egyptian oils before touching Cleopatra's beautiful skin.

You can use cream, full cream milk, buttermilk, goats' milk, or honey instead of the carrier oil.

A therapeutic bath can help to relieve aches and pains.

Make up the bath with up to 1 kg of Epsom salts and 6-8

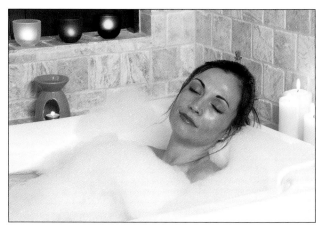

A bath reduces tension and anxiety

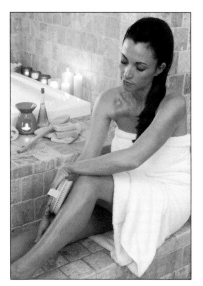

Dry body brush before your bath

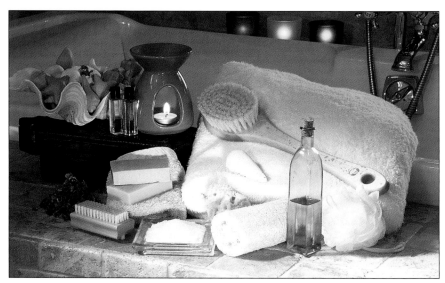

Be well prepared before you commence

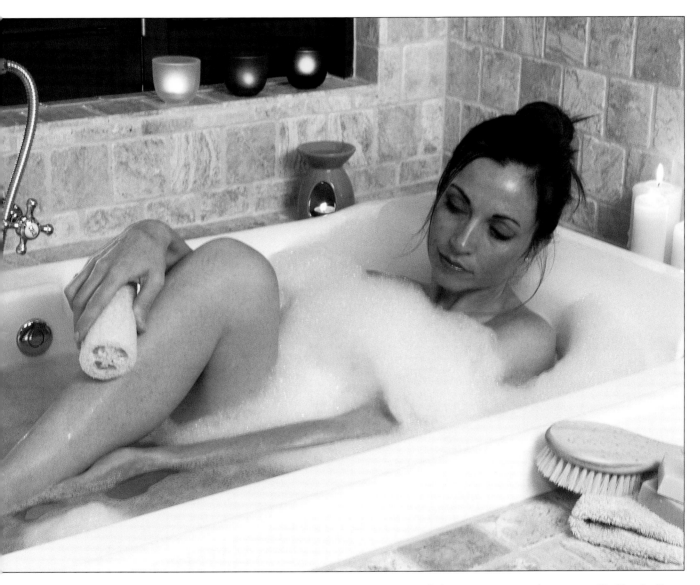

A bath is a pampering treat and promotes good health and wellbeing

drops of your chosen essential oils. Stay in the bath for 20 minutes. Then, dry well and lie flat on your bed, on a large, dry towel, covered with a towel and with another towel cushioning your neck and head. Cover yourself with a quilt and lie still for 20 minutes. Then complete the treatment with an ice-cold shower.

ESSENTIAL OILS IN WATER

(continued)

Other bath time suggestions

DIVINE BATH SALTS

- 1 cup Epsom salts (or ¹/₂ cup Epsom salts and ¹/₂ cup Dead Sea salt)

- 6–8 drops pure essential oil

- 2 drops glycerin

- 1 drop natural food colouring

Place all ingredients in stainless steel or glass bowl. Mix well and add to bath.

You can make up this recipe in larger amounts. Store in an airtight glass jar away from sunlight.

(Add only 1 cup per bath.)

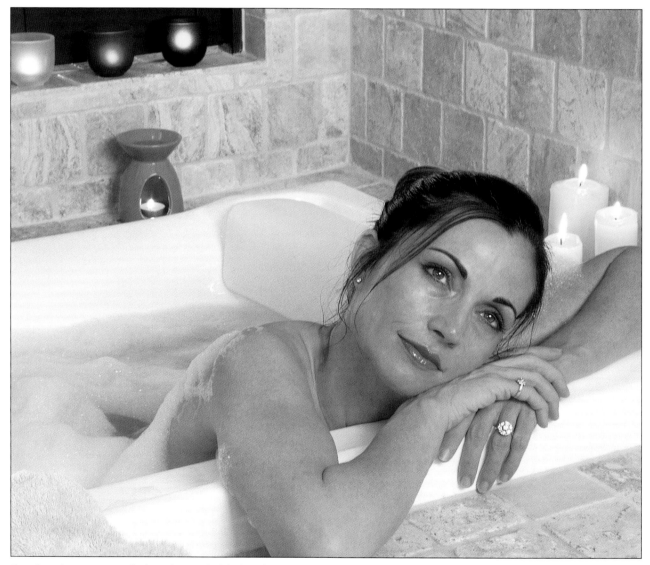

If you do not have any carrier oil, take a 'Cleopatra' bath for beautiful skin

FOOTBATH TREAT

So simple, yet so indulgent. This is especially good for tired, aching feet, but it will also lift the emotions, increase circulation and reduce perspiration.

- 2 tablespoons Epsom salts
- 1 dessertspoon carrier oil
- 4 drops of essential oil

Fill stainless or ceramic large bowl with water at the desired temperature, add salts and oils. Soak your feet for 15 minutes. For an extra treat, place a bag of marbles or smooth pebbles on the bottom of the basin whilst you are soaking and gently roll your feet back and forth. This gentle massage is like having a reflexology treatment. After the soak, massage the feet with an aromatic lotion, or dust the feet with an aromatic foot powder.

GIVING A FOOTBATH

Seat your friend in a comfortable chair. Place a large towel on the floor for subject's feet. Place a large bowl of water between their feet. Sit on the floor opposite on a cushion and place a second large towel on your legs to catch any spills.

1. Pick up one foot with your hand underneath it.
So you can check the temperature of the water as you submerge the foot. Follow with the other foot. Place your hands on their feet for a moment to connect with your subject.

2. Place your left hand under the arch of the left foot and your right hand supporting the ankle.
Slide your fingers in four large firm circular movements from heel to toes. Repeat three times.

3. Hold the left foot with both hands with thumbs on top and your fingers under the foot. Press your fingers into the arch of the foot, while your thumbs firmly stroke the top of the foot from the middle of the foot outwards, in four rhythmic movements. Work from the heel to the ball of the foot. Repeat three times.

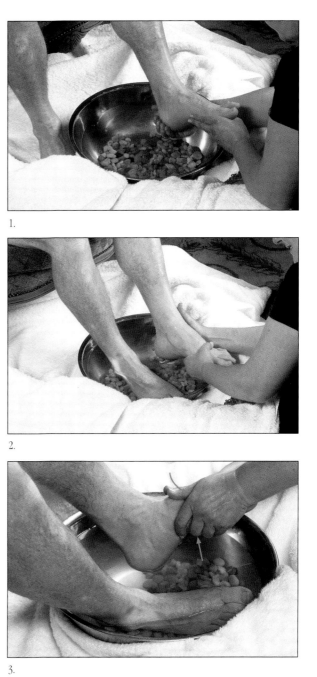

1.

2.

3.

4.

ESSENTIAL OILS IN WATER
(continued)

4. Rest right foot easily in bowl. Use both hands working in three circles, massage the Achilles tendon. Repeat three times.

5. With finger pads make small finger circles around each ankle three times.

6. Take a little water in both hands while your friend's foot still rests in bowl and wet the leg below the knee. Now firmly squeeze the calf muscle in four strong movements working down leg to the foot. Repeat three times.

7. Rest the outside of the left foot in the palm of your left hand. With the thumb of your right hand, work in five straight lines along the metatarsal bones from toes to ankle.

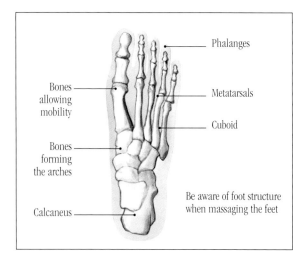

Phalanges

Bones allowing mobility

Metatarsals

Cuboid

Bones forming the arches

Calcaneus

Be aware of foot structure when massaging the feet

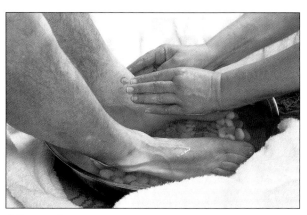

5. Finger circles

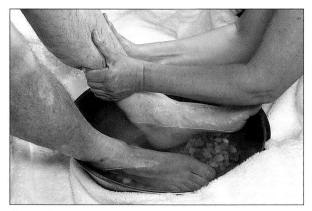

6 & 7. Calf massage

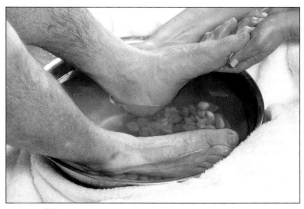

8. Twist off the toes

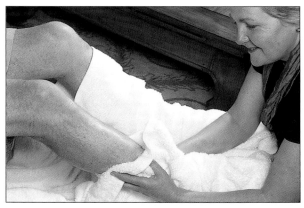

To finish, dry well

8. Retain the same hold and gently pull and twist each toe between your thumb and fingers of your right hand. Repeat steps 2-8 on the other foot.

Finally, rest both of your hands on their feet for a moment. Take one foot out at a time and rest them on your knees. Cover with the ends of the towel that is draped on your legs. Move the water bowl to the side. Draw your knees together and dry their legs and feet. Pay particular attention to drying firmly between each toe, dragging pointer finger and thumb from mid-foot to between the toes. Repeat three times.

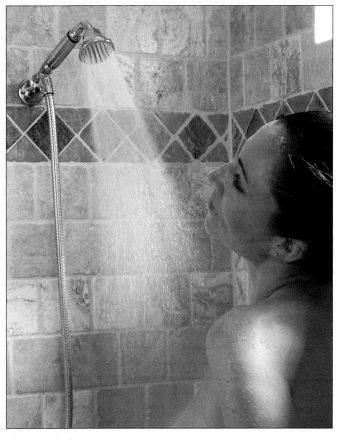
A shower can be therapeutic

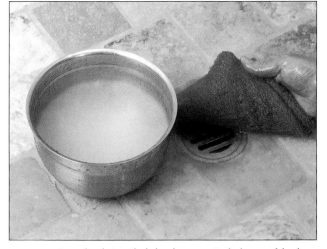
Cover plug drain with cloth to keep water in the bottom of the shower

SHOWER FOR PLEASURE

Cover the plug drain with a cloth to keep water in the bottom of the shower. Place 6–8 drops of your chosen essential oil in a pudding bowl and shower as usual. As the warm water splashes into the bowl, the aromas will diffuse so you inhale the therapeutic vapours. The bowl will overflow, allowing your feet to soak and absorb the oil's therapeutic benefits.

SUGGESTED OILS FOR BATH AND SHOWER TREATS

• For stimulation – basil and peppermint

• For relaxation – lavender and geranium

• For aching feet – thyme and chamomile

• For a cold bath – lemon and peppermint

• For a hot bath – ylang ylang and neroli

ESSENTIAL OILS IN WATER

(continued)

SAUNA

Add 3 drops of eucalyptus to the ladle of water you splash onto the coals, or 18 drops to the bucket of water. This makes a very pleasant inhalation.

SITZBATH

A large bowl or normal bath can be used, filled with enough water to cover your hips up to the waist. A cold bath, which you sit in for 3–5 minutes, offers great relief for bleeding in the middle of a cycle and for very heavy menstruation. It promotes sound sleep as well as being a preventative measure for colds and flu. A hot sitzbath is comforting for back pain, haemorrhoids, constipation and urinary problems.

COMPRESS

This is a great way to soothe aches and pains, relax spasms, cramps and swellings. A hot compress brings increased blood to the area to relieve congestion. Take a small bowl with 200 ml of water and add 10 drops of essential oil. Agitate the water. Fold a clean cloth or towel, immerse in the water, lightly squeeze out excess water and place on the area. Cover with a blanket or towel to maintain required temperature. When the cloth is at body temperature, reheat or cool as required. Repeat for up to four hours.

HOT COMPRESS For boils, splinters, abscesses, rheumatism, muscular pain, back ache, tummy ache, sore throat, chest congestion, toothache and menstrual cramps. Always test the hot compress before applying to be sure it is not too hot. A hot compress is excellent as a weekly hair treatment. Add 5 drops of pure essential oil to one tablespoon of carrier oil (such as avocado oil), massage into your scalp and follow with a hot towel compress.

Caution A hot compress should never be applied to swollen limbs.

COLD COMPRESS Ideal for sprains, bruises, headaches, burns, sunburn, chicken pox, hangovers, measles, high temperatures and to relieve inflammation. Leave the compress on for two to four hours. Must be kept moist (add ice blocks to the water).

WARM COMPRESS Good for skin treatments. When pure essential oils are used on the face in massage or an oil mask, the warm compress is used to infuse the oils into the skin.

Caution Avoid the eye area when administering a face compress.

HOT AND COLD COMPRESS Alternating hot and cold water is good for arthritis and infections.

STEAM INHALATION

Ideal for treating coughs and colds and for treating your skin to a steam facial. Place 1 litre of steaming hot water in a bowl. Add 5 drops of essential oil to the water. Bend forward over the bowl and drape a large towel over your head to trap the vapours. Inhale. Add some more boiling water to evaporate off any remaining essential oils.

GARGLE/MOUTHWASH A good way to treat halitosis, a sore throat or toothache. Add 2 drops of tea tree essential oil and 1 teaspoon of salt to a glass of warm water. Stir

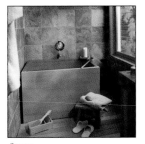
Sauna

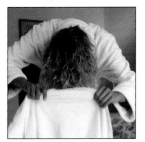
Compress

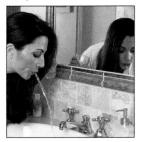
Gargle/mouthwash

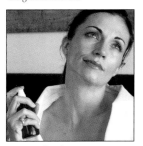
Spritz — facial spray

until salt is dissolved. Gargle every hour until symptoms are reduced. When gargling, keep the solution in the mouth/throat for as long as possible before spitting out. Do not swallow.

SPRITZ — FACIAL SPRAY

Floral waters are best made using de-ionized or distilled water. Most people use bottled spring water. Simply add 15 drops of essential oil to 50 ml of water. This is an excellent way to hydrate and freshen the skin, especially for office workers and travellers.

SPRITZ — AIR FRESHENER

Add 50 drops of essential oil to a 500 ml spray bottle for a natural, non-aerosol spray to deodorise, freshen and perfume a room.

SPRITZ — INSECT REPELLENT

Essential oils are an excellent, non-toxic way of beating an influx of insects. Mix 40 drops of essential oil to 100 ml of water. Use a pump spray bottle. Shake well before spraying into the air, onto your clothes or where insects scuttle.

LAUNDRY RINSE

Add 3 drops of essential oil to final rinse water.

SUGGESTED OILS

STEAM INHALATION
- Eucalyptus, peppermint, thyme, tea tree for chest, nasal and sinus problems.
- Lavender for headaches
- Sandalwood, frankincense, geranium for facial steams (use only 2 drops pure essential oil)

GARGLE/MOUTHWASH
- Tea tree, eucalyptus, vetiver, thyme and peppermint all contain compounds clinically proven to kill bacteria that cause bad breath, plaque and gum disease such as gingivitis.

Note: If you are suffering from toothache, make an appointment to see your dentist as soon as possible.

SPRITZ - FACIAL SPRAY
- For normal skin: Geranium and lavender
- For dry skin: Sandalwood and frankincense
- For oily skin: Cypress and lemon
- For blemished and sensitive skins: Chamomile and geranium

SPRITZ - AIR FRESHENER
- Lavender to kill airborne germs.
- Peppermint to remove the stale smell of cigarettes.
- Lemon or lime for cooking smells.
- Pine, rosemary or lavender for disinfecting.

SPRITZ - INSECT REPELLANT
- Camphor for moths.
- Citronella or lemongrass for mosquitoes and flying insects.
- Tea tree or peppermint for ants and fleas.
- Eucalyptus for cockroaches.

LAUNDRY RINSE
- Lemon and eucalyptus

ESSENTIAL OILS USED NEAT

Pure essential oil should not be used neat on the skin except in a few exceptional cases, but it can be used neat in many simple, highly effective ways around the home. Using neat on the skin: for a pimple, use lavender or tea tree oil on the end of a cotton bud; dab on to dry out, heal and ensure no infection. For cold sores do the same using rose geranium essential oil.

TISSUE INHALATION

Place 2 drops of essential oil on a tissue and place tissue in your cupped hand. Bend over whilst you empty your lungs with a big breath out. Take your hand to your nose and breathe in as you stand up and open your lung and abdominal areas. Repeat three times.

For the elderly or small children put the tissue in a simple paper funnel and perform the same routine. This dry inhalation can be used in many situations.

Suggested oils • Peppermint for uplifting and to keep awake on a long trip. • Lavender just before going to sleep. • Lemon or rosemary to stay focused when at work or studying.

TISSUE FOR SMELLY SHOES

Add 4 drops of essential oil to a tissue and immediately rub the entire sole of the shoe. Leave the tissue inside the shoe overnight.

Suggested oils • 2 drops each tea tree and lemon.

FOR INSOMNIA

Place one drop of essential oil on either side of a pillow to help insomnia.

Suggested oil • Lavender

FOR CONCENTRATION

Add one drop of oil to the page you are studying to assist your concentration.

Suggested oils • Rosemary, lemon, basil

AIR FRESHENER & INSECT REPELLENT

Add 2 drops of essential oil per cottonwool ball and place in cupboards, drawers, under fridge and stove as insect repellent. Place in air-conditioner vent and in vacuum cleaner to freshen the air.

Suggested oils • Eucalyptus, lemongrass or citronella as insect repellent or air freshener. • Lavender or geranium in your lingerie drawer.

CLEANING CLOTH

Add 4 drops directly to a damp cloth. Wipe surfaces inside cupboards, shelves and drawers, to disinfect, to clean, and to act as insect repellent.

Suggested oils • Combination of lavender, lemon, eucalyptus, geranium and tea tree.

WOOD FIRES

Add 2–3 drops of essential oil to each log and allow it to be absorbed into the wood. Add to fire as needed and enjoy the fragrance that it emits.

Suggested oils • Cedarwood, sandalwood, sweet orange, rose geranium, vetiver.

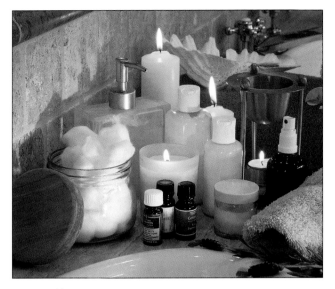
Creams and lotions

ESSENTIAL OILS IN UNSCENTED BASE CREAMS

Aromatherapy creams and lotions are easy to apply, they soothe and moisturise, are readily absorbed, protect and heal the skin and have a smooth non-greasy texture. The difference between a lotion and a cream is that with the lotion you add more water according to the consistency you prefer.

- Add 1 drop of essential oil to 2 ml of base cream for the body
- Add 1 drop of essential oil to 4 ml of base cream for the face

Select the essential oil according to the condition you are treating. Store your lotion or cream in a sealed glass jar in a cool place.

ESSENTIAL OILS IN POWDER

Body and foot powders are used to scent, deodorise and disinfect the skin. To make your own powders measure the amount of rice/cornflour needed and pour into a small, wide-mouthed jar, then add the essential oils. Mix ingredients thoroughly. Allow the powder to stand for a day or two before use.

FOR ITCHY SKIN

- 5 drops each of patchouli, lime, chamomile and lavender oil
- 1 cup cornflour

AROMATIC FOOT POWDER

- 6 drops each of lemongrass, petitgrain, tea tree and lavender essential oil
- 2 tablespoons cornflour

Dust in shoes, on socks and sprinkle on blisters for rapid healing – .and no more smelly feet!

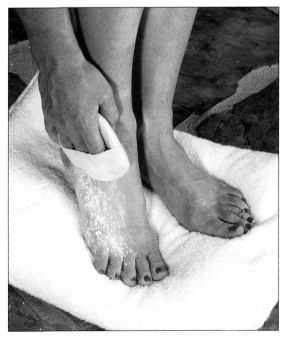
No more smelly feet!

ESSENTIAL OILS IN PURE ALCOHOL

You can blend essential oils with alcohol to create a perfume that is just for you.

The essential oils must be used undiluted. The water should be distilled or bottled spring water. Ideally you should use pure pharmaceutical alcohol, but this is only available in Europe. Vodka is suitable however; use the highest proof you can obtain. Do make a note of your formulations in drops. The strength of perfume can vary depending on the ratio of essential oil to water and alcohol.

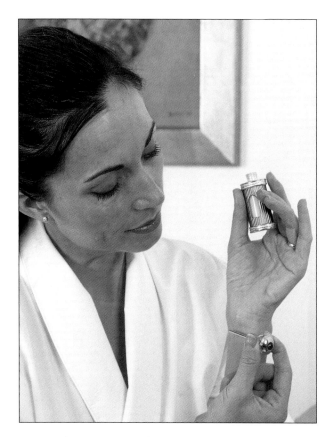

Create a perfume that's just right for you

EAU DE TOILETTE

- 5 drops each of rosemary, basil and petitgrain oil
- 10 drops each of bergamot, lemon and neroli oil
- 15 drops of orange oil
- 70 ml vodka
- 30 ml spring water

Add the essential oils to vodka in a glass bottle with a screw top. Stir well and leave it to stand for 48 hours. Now add spring water. Stir well and leave to stand for a further 48 hours. By leaving the formula to mature for 4–6 weeks, the fragrance will be even stronger. Filter it through a coffee filter and bottle.

PERFUME

To make a perfume, choose from the following, balancing the scents to create your own distinctive fragrance.

- 75 drops in total from the following pure essential oils: cedarwood, clary sage, geranium, lavender, lemon, lemongrass, lime, marjoram, neroli, sandalwood, vetiver
- 20 ml vodka
- 5 ml spring water

Add 75 drops in total of essential oils listed above to vodka. Shake well. Leave to stand for 48 hours. Now add spring water. Shake well. Leave for 4–6 weeks for the synergy to be complete.

USING ESSENTIAL OILS

	APPLICATIONS	ESSENTIAL OIL	
carrier oils	*Massage *Friction rub *Pulse point *Chest rub	Body – 1 drop in 2 ml carrier oil Face – 1 drop in 4 ml carrier oil 1 drop in 1 ml carrier oil 1 drop in 1 ml carrier oil Body – 1 drop in 2 ml cream/lotion Face – 1 drop in 4 ml cream/lotion	CARRIER OILS
Air	Essential oil warmers Saucer/water bowl Light bulb Car fragrancing candles	6–8 drops in water for a candle warmer or saucer of water 6–8 drops directly for electric warmer 6–8 drops 1–2 drops on a light bulb ring	AIR
water	*Bath *Bath salts *Foot/hand/sitz bath *Shower *Douche *Steam inhalation *Compress Air freshener spray *Facial spray Insect spray *Gargle/mouth wash Laundry wash Jacuzzi	6–8 drops in a full bath 6–8 drops added to Epsom salts/Dead Sea salt 4 drops in a bowl of water 6 drops in a bowl and place in shower 5–10 drops, 1 teaspoon cider vinegar in 1 litre of water 2–3 drops in a bowl of steaming water. Cover with towel 10 drops in 1 litre cold/hot water. Soak cloth and place directly on skin and cover 25 drops in 100 ml of water in a spray bottle 5 drops in 20 ml of spring water in spray bottle 40 drops in 100 ml spray bottle 1–2 drops, 1 teaspoon of salt in a small glass of boiled warm water 3 drops in final rinse/fabric softener section 3 drops per person	WATER
neat	Tissue Paper funnel Pillow Cotton wool balls Curtain Cleaning cloth Candle Wood fires	2 drops on tissue 2 drops on tissue inserted in paper funnel 1 drop on either side of pillow 3 drops per ball 2 drops directly on hem at regular intervals 4 drops neat on damp cloth. Wear gloves. 2–3 drops 1–2 drops per log	NEAT
unscented base creams	Creams & Lotions	Body – 1 drop in 2 ml cream/lotion Face – 1 drop in 4 ml cream/lotion	UNSCENTED BASE CREAMS
powder	*Body powder *Foot powder	20 drops to 1 cup rice flour/cornflour 6 drops to 2 tablespoons rice flour/cornflour	POWDER
alcohol	*Eau de toilette *Perfume	60 drops to 70 ml vodka to 30 ml spring water 75 drops to 20 ml vodka to 5 ml spring water	ALCOHOL

* You may use half the adult dosage for children and the elderly. For babies, you may use a quarter

of the adult dosage but only those oils recommended for babies.

Note: For additional information related to expectant mothers and children, see p 74 – 75.

WHICH OIL TO USE?

TREATMENTS	ESSENTIAL OILS
Anti-bacterial	Lime, tea tree, thyme, lavender, cypress, rosemary, eucalyptus
Antidepressant	Melissa, jasmine, grapefruit, patchouli, orange, rose, ylang ylang, clary sage, basil, patchouli, petitgrain, rose, bergamot
Anti-fungal	Lemongrass, lime, tea tree, lavender
Anti-inflammatory	Bergamot, chamomile, lavender
Anti-microbial	Tea tree, bergamot, chamomile
Antiseptic	Bergamot, eucalyptus, lime, lavender, tea tee
Anti-viral	Tee tree, eucalyptus, fennel, ginger, juniper, bergamot, lemon, cedarwood, jasmine, lime, mandarin, neroli, patchouli, peppermint, pine, rose, rosewood, sandalwood, thyme, vetiver, juniper
Aphrodisiac	Clary sage, jasmine, neroli, rosewood, sandalwood, vetiver, ylang ylang
Astringent	Juniper, cedarwood, cypress, lemongrass, lime, rose, sandalwood, eucalyptus
Calming	Fennel, juniper, lavender, mandarin, melissa, marjoram, sandalwood
Concentration aid	Lemon, rosemary, basil
Deodorant	Lavender, neroli, orange
De-stressing	Petitgrain, lemongrass, rosewood, eucalyptus, patchouli, bergamot
Detoxifier	Fennel, juniper, lemon, rosemary
Digestive	Mandarin, peppermint, marjoram, orange, chamomile, ginger
Disinfectant	Lime, pine, lemon
Diuretic	Juniper, lemon, mandarin, sandalwood, eucalyptus, thyme, fennel, rosemary

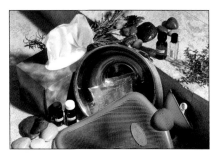
First aid kit

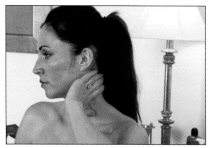
Self massage

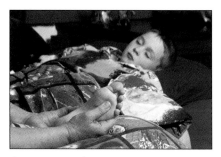
Foot massage to relax

TREATMENTS	ESSENTIAL OILS
Energising	Basil, rosemary, peppermint, lemon
Expectorant	Marjoram, tea tree, eucalyptus, frankincense, lavender, peppermint
Insect repellent	Eucalyptus, lemongrass, lemon, cedarwood, rosemary, tea tree
Lowers blood pressure	Lavender, marjoram, melissa, ylang ylang
Nerve relaxant	Melissa, clary sage, neroli, orange, eucalyptus, vetiver, basil, marjoram
Pain reliever	Bergamot, chamomile (roman), peppermint, eucalyptus, lavender, rosemary
Raises blood pressure	Clary sage, peppermint, rosemary
Reduces fever	Bergamot, chamomile, eucalyptus, lavender, peppermint, tea tree
Relieves flatulence	Petitgrain, peppermint, ginger, lavender, chamomile
Relieves insomnia	Neroli, lavender, chamomile
Sedative and relaxing	Cedarwood, lavender, mandarin, marjoram, frankincense, vetiver, chamomile (roman), jasmine, melissa, patchouli, rose, rosewood, ylang ylang
Stimulant	Eucalyptus, rosemary, lemon, peppermint, fennel, eucalyptus, thyme, tea tree, basil, bergamot, cypress
Strengthens body's immune system	Lavender, eucalyptus, rosewood, tea tree
Tonic	Mandarin, melissa, grapefruit, rosemary, sandalwood, thyme, vetiver, basil, bergamot, geranium, ginger, lavender, tea tree
Uplifting and refreshing	Basil, peppermint, rosemary, lemon, bergamot, rose geranium, lavender, melissa, orange, pine
Warming	Marjoram, ginger
Wound healing	Lavender, chamomile, geranium, rosemary, tea tree, bergamot

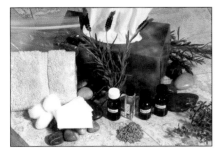

Travel kit

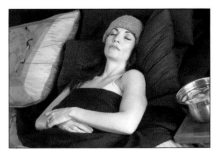

Compress to relieve headaches

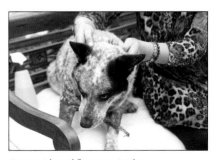

Prevent ticks and fleas on animals

PREGNANCY

What a beautiful time for a woman to indulge. This is an important time for mother and baby to be as healthy as possible. After the first four months of the pregnancy, essential oils can be used to enhance the feeling of wellbeing.

During pregnancy, the body changes are so rapid that after the first four months, the benefits of aromatherapy massage are enormous, both physically and emotionally.

STRETCH MARKS

Pregnancy massage oil • 25 ml jojoba, vitamin E and wheatgerm carrier oil (use only carrier oil in first four months) • 3 drops lavender • 3 drops frankincense • 3 drops sandalwood • 3 drops bergamot

Upper thighs: massage twice daily with firm upward strokes.

Tummy: massage twice daily, using only light circular strokes, in a clockwise direction, pinching to encourage elasticity of the skin

MORNING SICKNESS AND FAINTING

Always carry a tissue with you and have lavender and peppermint essential oils with you.

Add 2 drops to a tissue and inhale deeply. Repeat till you feel better.

NOTE: THE FOLLOWING OILS SHOULD NOT BE USED DURING PREGNANCY

basil, cedarwood, clary sage, clove bud, cypress, fennel, jasmine, juniper, lemongrass, marjoram, peppermint, rosemary, thyme.

BABY AND CHILD CARE

Aromatherapy is invaluable when caring for young children. Careful use of pure, natural essential oils provides a natural alternative to chemical drugs. Essential oils can be used for everyday common ailments and as a complementary treatment for general wellbeing. They are not intended to replace the health care practitioner, however, and for any serious or ongoing condition a professional should be consulted.

Children from as young as 48 hours old can be gently massaged daily using lavender and chamomile oils. This will help bond mother and baby and ensure security and stability. Use the same soothing music at bathtime when you massage. Be sure the environment is warm. Apricot kernel or jojoba carrier oil is very nourishing for young skin. For the bath, use 1 drop of lavender oil in 1 teaspoon of carrier oil. For massage, blend 1 drop of lavender or chamomile oil to 10 ml of carrier oil. These two oils calm the nervous system.

3 months –1 year old: calendula, tea tree and grapefruit can be added to essential oils safe to use on baby

1–5 years: geranium, lemon, palmarosa and rose can be added

5–12 years: all oils considered safe for adults, but using one quarter of the adult dosage

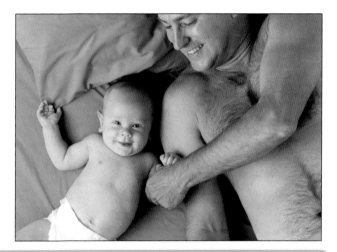

COLIC
(1 drop of lavender and 1 drop of geranium oil in 15 ml carrier oil)
• Use as a compress on tummy, or massage on tummy in a gentle clockwise direction.

CRADLE CAP
(1 drop of geranium and 1 drop of eucalyptus oil in 15 ml avocado carrier oil)
• Massage into scalp in morning and leave on all day. Wash at bath time and gently lift any loose pieces. Repeat daily till the scalp is clear.

HEAT RASH
(2 drops of lavender oil added to 1 litre of cooled chamomile tea)
• Bathe as required.

NAPPY RASH
(1 drop each of lavender and chamomile oil to 20 ml of calendula oil)
• Apply the blend at every nappy change till completely healed.
Also, take care to wash and dry well after each nappy change. Be very careful of using powders with mineral oils; they clog the skin. Avoid plastic pants and disposable nappies as they discourage air circulation and retain body heat and moisture.

TEETHING
(1 drop each of lavender and chamomile essential oil in 20 ml carrier oil)
• Gently apply to jawline, upper neck and cheeks as often as is necessary.

ROOM SPRAY
• You can use an air spray in the room once the infant is over one year old. Use one quarter of the adult dose.

COUGHS AND COLDS
(Add 3 drops of tea tree or lavender oil to a bowl of boiling water)
• Place the bowl under baby's cot. Use lavender and tea tree massage oil as a chest and back rub.

INSECT BITES/BURNS
(1 drop of lavender oil in 1 teaspoon of bicarbonate of soda. Mix the oil and bicarb into a paste with cold water).
• Apply as often as necessary.

CALMING BATH
(1 teaspoon sweet almond carrier oil, 1 drop each of lavender and mandarin oils)
• Put the oils into a warm bath. Allow your child to lie still as you gently massage their limbs. Play calming music.

INSOMNIA
A warm bath to soothe, followed by a warm drink of chamomile tea whilst you read them their favourite story. Use 1 drop of chamomile/geranium/lavender/mandarin oil on each side of their pillow. Massage under their feet with 1 drop of oil in 1 teaspoon sweet almond/grapeseed carrier oil. Last of all a great big gentle hug followed by light butterfly kisses.

TREATING COMMON AILMENTS

Essential oils assist the body to heal itself by lowering stress levels, relaxing and toning the muscles, stimulating the immune system, the organs and the glands in the body to fight bacteria, fungi and viruses. These oils can be used to relieve symptoms and help the natural healing of common, everyday ailments. I hope you will enjoy using these simple and relatively inexpensive methods to enrich your friends' and family's health and wellbeing. See the reference chart for common ailments, showing which oils to choose and the application method suggested. Be sure you are familiar with the application method (see page 71). Essential oils must be used in the correct way and the correct dilution as misuse can cause toxicity.

Be sure that you are only treating common problems. If symptoms are severe, or continue, please seek consultation with your naturopath or health care professional.

Before preparing the remedy, check the Guidelines When Using Essential Oils (page 8) as well as the cautions on the specific oil you are about to use.

COMPLEMENTARY THERAPY

Aromatherapy is a complementary therapy and needs to go hand-in-hand with the following lifestyle checks to be fully effective:

- Diet correction
- Regular exercise
- Drink 2 litres of water per day, every day
- Cut coffee completely from your diet
- Reduce alcohol consumption to a maximum of two glasses five days a week for women, and three glasses five days a week for men – every week of the year.
- Have enough quality sleep every day, week after week.
  The optimum is in bed and asleep by 10.00 pm. Up at 6.00 am.
- Reduce stress wherever possible.

Last, but by no means least, correct the balance in your life between work life, home life and spiritual life, and include time for relaxation.

With all the above in place and aromatherapy at work there will be strides made. Have fun on the path of love, light and laughter with aromatherapy your constant companion.

Treatments - Abbreviations

aM	Abdomen massage
B	Bath
C	Compress
cC	Cold compress
cM	Chest massage
CR	Cream
CWB	Cottonwool balls
fB	Footbath
FM	Face massage
fR	Friction rub massage
hB	Hand bath
hC	Hot compress
h&cC	Hot and cold compress
h&fB	Hand and footbath
h&fM	Hand and foot massage
hG	Hot gargle/mouthwash
icC	Ice cold compress
L	Lotion
M	Massage
N	Neat
P	Perfume
PP	Pulse point massage
rS	Room spray
SB	Skin brushing
sB	Sitz bath
sI	Steam inhalation
sM	Scalp massage
sS	Spritz facial spray
ThB	Therapeutic bath
tI	Tissue inhalation

ESSENTIAL OILS FOR COMMON AILMENTS

Common Ailments	Helpful Pure Essential Oil	Method of Application
Abdominal pain	Peppermint, chamomile, marjoram, fennel	M B
Abscesses	Lavender, tea tree, chamomile	hC
Dental abscess	Tea tree, lavender	hG
Acne	Patchouli, lavender, roman chamomile, geranium	FM
Arthritis and rheumatism	Cypress, fennel, lemon, ginger, frankincense, eucalyptus, pine, lavender, pine, rosemary	ThB sI M h&tC
Athletes foot	Tea tree, lavender, geranium, patchouli	fB
Anxiety and stress	Basil, sandalwood, bergamot, frankincense, cypress, lavender, neroli, patchouli, orange, rose	B M tI P PP
Bruises	Lavender, fennel, geranium, cypress	M icC
Black eye	Lavender	cC
Bleeding (external)	Geranium, lemon, chamomile, cypress	icC
Blisters	Chamomile, lavender	N sS icC
Bilious attack	Rosemary, fennel	N
Backache	Chamomile, lavender and frankincense	M B
Bunions	Chamomile, melissa, peppermint, lavender, cypress, lemon	fB M h&tC
Burns	Lavender	N sS icC
Broken capillaries	Chamomile, cypress, rose, lavender, lemon	B M C
Chapped lips	Chamomile, geranium	CR
Cystitis	Sandalwood, bergamot, tea tree	aM sB
Cellulite	Cypress, lavender, fennel, geranium, grapefruit, rosemary	M SB
Circulation and chilblains	Cypress, ginger, rosemary, marjoram, eucalyptus, geranium, lavender	h&fB h&fM
Colds and flu	Lemon, eucalyptus, tea tree, pine, thyme	ThB rS tI sI
Coldsore (herpes)	Melissa, bergamot, geranium, lavender, tea tree and patchouli	N C L
Constipation & digestive problems	Rosemary, lemon, peppermint, lemongrass, orange (slow digestion)	C aM
Corns	Lemon	N
Coughs	Eucalyptus, thyme	sI cM
Dandruff	Cedarwood, lavender, rosemary, geranium, tea tree, sandalwood	hC sM
Dermatitis and psoriasis	Frankincense, chamomile, geranium, lavender, rosewood and bergamot	B M C L CR
Diarrhoea	Peppermint, eucalyptus, chamomile, tea tree, lavender, geranium	aM
Earache	Chamomile, lavender, tea tree	CWB
Eczema (dry)	Chamomile, geranium, patchouli	B M C L CR
Eczema (weeping)	Bergamot, juniper, melissa	B C L CR
Fatigue	Geranium, peppermint, rosemary, basil, clary sage	B fB tI
Foot blisters	Chamomile, lavender, tea tree	N
Fluid retention	Cypress, fennel, grapefruit, juniper, geranium, bergamot	C L ThB
Fungal Infection (eg: tinea)	Geranium, lemongrass, tea tree, lavender, patchouli	hB P L C
Haemorrhoids	Patchouli, geranium, chamomile	C sB
Hair loss	Lavender, rosemary, clary sage, ylang ylang	sM
Halitosis	Peppermint, lemon, tea tree, lavender and thyme	hG
Hay Fever	Chamomile, lemon, lavender	sI P PP
Headaches	Lavender, lemongrass, marjoram, peppermint, rose, rosewood, vetiver	P PP
Hiccups	Lavender, lemon	fR tI M *(throat, solar plexus and abdomen)*
High blood pressure	Lemon	M
Indigestion	Peppermint, ginger, lemongrass	aM
Insomnia	Lavender, orange, lemon, mandarin, rose, sandalwood, vetiver, ylang ylang, geranium, neroli, jasmine	tI M B
Itching skin	Chamomile, cedarwood, bergamot, lavender, patchouli, lime	B M L
Mosquito repellent	Eucalyptus, peppermint, citronella, geranium	rS L
Muscular aches	Rosemary, eucalyptus, basil, lavender, clary sage	M B C
Muscular stiffness	Rosemary, neroli, melissa, cypress, peppermint	M B C
Muscular tone	Lavender, lemongrass, marjoram, neroli	M B C
Nausea	Peppermint, basil, fennel, ginger	M sI
PMT	Clary sage, orange, lemon, chamomile, geranium, neroli, mandarin	M B
Respiratory congestion	Rosemary, eucalyptus, frankincense, pine, chamomile, patchouli	M tI
Smelly feet	Cedarwood, cypress, citronella	P fB CWB *(in shoes)*
Sinusitis	Rosemary, eucalyptus, peppermint, lemon, pine	sI P PP
Shingles	Geranium, bergamot, chamomile	N C
Snoring	Thyme	fR
Sprains	Eucalyptus, chamomile, lavender	C
Sore throat	Eucalyptus, lime, tea tree, thyme, frankincense	sI M hG *(throat and neck)*
Sunburn	Lavender, peppermint, tea tree, chamomile	sS cC *(on head)*
Toothache	Chamomile, lemon, peppermint, tea tree	hG
Varicose veins	Cypress, lemon, rosemary, lavender, geranium	M C B
Warts	Lemon, lavender	N

BEAUTY AND SKIN CARE

A healthy, glowing skin is the basis for looking and feeling great. Using natural products with essential oils, which have nourishing and healing properties that penetrate the skin, you are on the way to healthier younger-looking skin. Enjoy being creative with the suggested essential oils, using the recipe for facial sprays, creams and lotions.

ESSENTIAL OILS FOR SKIN CARE

SKIN TYPE	ESSENTIAL & CARRIER OILS
Sensitive	• Lavender, sandalwood, chamomile • Carrier oil for cleansing – grape seed oil and apricot seed • Rosewater for toning
Blemished	• Geranium, lavender, patchouli • Carrier oil – grape seed and evening primrose • Rosewater for toning
Mature	• Frankincense, ylang ylang, sandalwood, chamomile • Carrier oil – rosehip oil and evening primrose • Rosewater for toning
Oily	• Bergamot, lemon, cypress, sandalwood • Carrier oil – sweet almond oil and wheat germ • Witch-hazel for toning
Combination	• Sandalwood, ylang ylang, rosewood and lavender • Carrier oil – sweet almond oil and evening primrose • Witch-hazel for toning
Dry	• Rosewood, ylang ylang, patchouli, rose • Carrier oil – avocado oil and jojoba • Rosewater for toning
Normal	• Palmarosa, lavender, geranium and ylang ylang • Carrier oil – sweet almond oil and evening primrose • Witch-hazel for toning

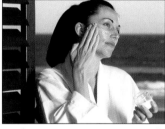
Facial creams

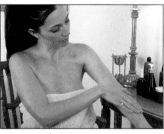
Moisturising body lotion

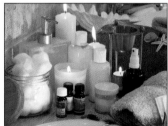
A variety of beauty products

Enjoy being creative with these suggested essential oils, using the recipe for facial sprays, creams and lotions.

Cleansing: Use sweet almond oil for a facial massage. Press with tissue to remove then use toner to remove surplus oil.

Toning: Toning gently stimulates the circulation, restoring the skin's natural acid balance, leaving it feeling fresh and clean. Add 6 drops of chosen essential oil to ¹/₂ cup toner (select both from chart above) ¹/₂ cup spring water and 2 teaspoons cider vinegar. Leave for 3–4 days to synergise. Shake well before use.

Facial steaming: This causes the skin to perspire, helping to loosen grime and dead skin cells.

The heat increases the blood supply to the surface of the skin to assist hydration, giving it a more youthful, softer tone. For facial steam, prepare as for steam inhalation, choosing oils from above list.

ABOUT THE AUTHOR

MARGIE HARE was born in Cape Town, South Africa. She was a speech and drama teacher then a publishing sales executive before establishing her own business specialising in growing and marketing herbs. An intense interest in the therapeutic power of herbs led Margie to study other alternative-healing therapies, including aromatherapy, reflexology and massage. In 1994, she won the prestigious Herb Woman of the Year award for education in the field of herbs and healing. During this time, she was herb consultant and lecturer at one of South Africa's leading health resorts, Stellenbosch Hydro. In 1996, Margie moved to Australia as a marketing executive with a wine company, but was soon managing her own alternative-health business, Divine Touch. She now practises as a holistic healing therapist in aromatherapy, reflexology, Dr Vodder Manual Lymph Drainage and combined decongestive therapy, remedial massage, reike and crystal point therapy. Margie is also a consultant and lecturer at Hopewood Health Centre, one of Australia's top health retreats. She is a member of the Australasian Vodder Therapists Association (AVTA) and Remedial Masseurs Association (RMA), and president of the North Sydney chapter of Business Network International, a global business-marketing organisation.

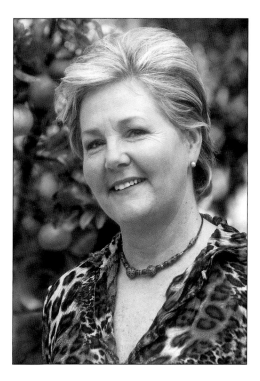

Divine Touch

"Massage tailored to balance your body"

www.divinearomatherapy.com.au

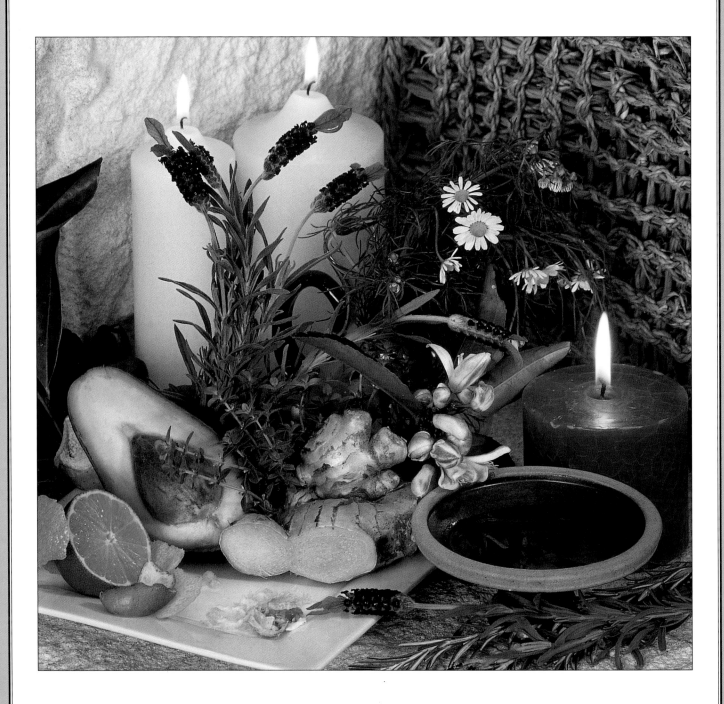